"Severe Trauma and Stress Recovery: Techniques and What it Takes to Thrive is a rare bridge between clinical sensitivity and operational clarity—highly recommended for practitioners and survivors alike.

From 2008 onward, at our Institute, we have tested many of the methods in the first edition of this handbook (*What it Takes to Thrive: Techniques for Severe Trauma and Stress Recovery*) across our therapy training programmes—now well over a thousand students.

John Henden has been a valued recurring guest teacher, and the approach proves consistently practical and teachable.

Follow-up with trainees confirms the techniques translate reliably into real client work, especially where severe stress narrows hope and options.

—John Pihlaja MSc Solution Focused Therapy,
Chartered Psychologist, AFBPsS
CEO, Helsinki Psychotherapy Institute, Finland
www.psykoterapiakoulutus.fi

"John Henden delivers a practical guide filled with helpful, straightforward, and effective tools to aid recovery from the impacts of severe stress and trauma. These are born out years of experience in the field, as well as in the research literature, on what is *actually* helpful. Survivors are able to use this resource in a workbook style, and it is also accessible to professionals looking for a resource to support their work."

—Dr. James Brown
Clinical Psychologist and Lecturer – University of New England,
NSW, Australia

Severe Trauma and Stress Recovery: Techniques and What it Takes to Thrive is not a book that gathers dust on a bookshelf. It is a handbook full of solid and proven to be successful strategies and tools to encourage, support and empower survivors of severe trauma and stress; as well as providing practitioners with life changing tools and strategies they can implement with confidence.

The content of this book changes lives and offers hope, with John Henden's own insights and experiences woven throughout the pages. It is a 'must have' for all living with or working with, those impacted by trauma and stress."

—Caroline Loo, BSS, MNZAC
Director, Invercargill Loss and Grief Centre,
New Zealand

"John Henden, a leading figure in Solution-Focused Brief Therapy, has authored practical books that have been widely translated internationally, including in ethnic-Chinese cultural regions. This book comprehensively presents his extensive practical experience and years of training expertise. The effective knowledge and specific operational steps presented in the book, imbued with wisdom and compassion, greatly assist trauma survivors thrive in adversity. For practitioners, it is an invaluable professional handbook for applying solution-focused approaches in trauma recovery work."

—Dr. Hsu Wei-Su
Retired Professor, Department of Educational Psychology and
Counseling, National Taiwan Normal University, Taiwan
Honorary Advisor, Taiwan Solution-Focused Center
SFBT trainer in ethnic-Chinese cultural regions

"John Henden's book offers readers who are looking for help something extremely important: hope. Hope contained in descriptions of coping and using specific tools presented in the book by other people—clients who have gone through trauma and coped with it. This is a gift that cannot be overestimated.

John Henden also addresses professionals and others who accompany people in coping with trauma with a message about retraumatization and revictimization.

This book helps people to build a new and better life; to become a person who lives life to the fullest; and a person who has not been stopped by what they unfortunately had to experience. That should be the goal, shouldn't it?

John Henden's book helps us achieve this. I encourage you to read it."

—**Jacek Lelonkiewicz**
CEO, Centrum Terapii Krótkoterminowej
Łódź, Poland
https://www.centrumtk.com/

"Books and treatments for trauma too often focus on simply reducing symptoms. While this is welcome, John Henden goes much further, emphasizing thriving and finding solutions. The very nature of Solution-Focused Therapy is inspiring, and Henden is a master of awakening individuals' capacities to thrive and flourish. Even beyond this, he has expertly crafted this book to be equally helpful to survivors and practitioners alike. And to top it off, the publisher has ensured that this book is presented in the most user-friendly way possible. In an era of dwindling resources and a lack of expertise, this book is all the more necessary."

—David Prescott
Director, Safer Society Continuing Education Center
Vermont, USA
www.safersociety.org

"John Henden approaches the emotive and disturbing arena of severe trauma with a lightness of touch and an eye for very practical and usable techniques, easily applicable for both sufferer or practitioner to try out. He brings his long experience of working in NHS Mental Health Services in England together with a broad knowledge of Solution Focussed Therapy, in which he is an internationally known trainer. This approach to therapy and counselling is an important contribution, especially in its application to combat stress and PTSD. It forms the basis of this excellent, newly expanded and updated, self-help book."

—Professor Harry Procter
University of Hertfordshire, UK

SEVERE TRAUMA
AND
STRESS RECOVERY

Techniques and What it Takes to Thrive

SEVERE TRAUMA

AND

STRESS RECOVERY

Techniques and What it Takes to Thrive

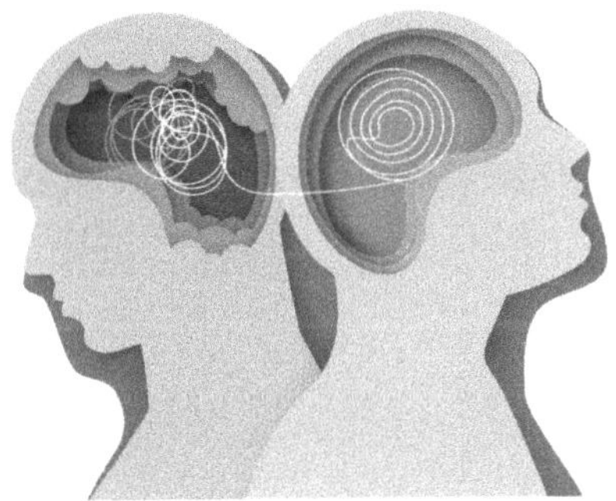

John Henden

John Henden Consultancy Ltd, UK

World Scientific

NEW JERSEY · LONDON · SINGAPORE · BEIJING · SHANGHAI · HONG KONG · TAIPEI · CHENNAI · TOKYO

Published by

World Scientific Publishing Co. Pte. Ltd.

5 Toh Tuck Link, Singapore 596224

USA office: 27 Warren Street, Suite 401-402, Hackensack, NJ 07601

UK office: 57 Shelton Street, Covent Garden, London WC2H 9HE

Library of Congress Cataloging-in-Publication Data

Names: Henden, John author

Title: Severe trauma and stress recovery : techniques and what it takes to thrive /
    John Henden, John Henden Consultancy Ltd, UK.

Other titles: What it takes to thrive

Description: [New edition]. | New Jersey : World Scientific, [2026] |
    Original title: What it takes to thrive: techniques for severe trauma and stress recovery. |
    Includes bibliographical references and index. |
    Audience: Ages Any age | Audience: Grades 10-12

Identifiers: LCCN 2026001705 (print) | LCCN 2026001706 (ebook) |
    ISBN 9789819814008 hardcover | ISBN 9789819814824 paperback |
    ISBN 9789819814015 ebook | ISBN 9789819814022 ebook

Subjects: LCSH: Post-traumatic stress disorder--Treatment | Psychic trauma--Treatment

Classification: LCC RC552.P67 H453 2026 (print) | LCC RC552.P67 (ebook)

LC record available at https://lccn.loc.gov/2026001705

LC ebook record available at https://lccn.loc.gov/2026001706

British Library Cataloguing-in-Publication Data

A catalogue record for this book is available from the British Library.

For any available supplementary material, please visit
https://www.worldscientific.com/worldscibooks/10.1142/14338#t=suppl

Desk Editor: Geysilla Jean Ortiz
Cover design: Loo Chuan Ming

Project managed and typeset by Manila Typesetting Company (MTC)

Dedication

I dedicate this book to the many survivors I have known and met—especially at training workshops and conferences—who have shown remarkable determination to reach the "thriver" stage of their journey. Despite the severity of traumatic events they may have experienced, whether in childhood or adulthood, they have chosen to live life to the fullest, and in many cases, have gone on to achieve great things. They are shining examples of what is possible and serve as a great encouragement to others who are still at earlier stages in their healing journey.

I also dedicate this book to the many severe trauma recovery clients I have had the privilege to work with over the past 30 years. They have taught me so much about their innovative and idiosyncratic ways of overcoming their post-trauma experiences. I expect their stories to continue to inspire not only my present and future clients, but also the participants of the workshops I lead.

Disclaimer

This book has been written and published for informational purposes and is not intended to serve as a substitute for professional therapy or treatment for any specific condition or complaint. While the author and publisher aim to provide valuable information and advice for consideration, it is ultimately up to each survivor—as well as their spouse, partner, buddy, or family member—to seek out and find whatever works best for them.

The Book's Purpose

As both a therapist and a trainer, I have spent over 30 years working with individuals affected by severe trauma and stress. Throughout this time, I have noted the dire shortage of appropriate, skilled support for those in need. In many cases, even when help was available, it was either the wrong kind of help and/or the practitioner's skills have been insufficient.

Many publications have been designed to provide help for survivors of severe trauma and stress. Only few, however, provide practical, specific tips and techniques for recovery.

Many textbooks aimed at helping practitioners tend to concentrate more on background information—awareness, demographics, personality factors, and statistics—rather than getting down to specifics of what truly works. Even those that include tools and techniques only describe few or explain them in an overly complex and technical way, appealing mainly to academic practitioners. This comprehensive guide, offering a wide range of tools and techniques, aims to fill this gap in provision.

This book has been carefully designed to support both survivors and practitioners.

It should be emphasised that most people who experience traumatic life events are able to return to relative normality within a few days or weeks, after talking about it with relatives and friends, or by mentally processing it on their own. However, it is the 15%–20% who experience a longer, more pronounced reaction who may benefit most from this book.

Psychotherapists, counsellors, welfare workers, and lay workers with a heart for working with survivors of severe trauma and stress will find all they need within this book. It is divided into six sections: triggers, flashbacks, intrusive thoughts, sleep disturbance, "the lows", and living life to the full.

Most of the more than 130 tools and techniques included in this book are easy to understand and apply— both by survivors of severe trauma and stress, and by therapists and counsellors. For welfare and lay workers, a basic counselling skills qualification is recommended. It is a one-stop-shop handbook for both survivors and practitioners.

An overriding hope in writing this book is to encourage more practitioners to work in the field of severe trauma and stress recovery. As the well-known saying goes, "The harvest is plentiful but the workers are few."

Many avoid working with survivors of severe trauma for the following reasons:

- Fear of saying something that might unintentionally make the person feel worse
- Fear of hearing something that could potentially be traumatising
- The mistaken belief that there are "thousands of experts out there" just waiting to take the referral

Most survivors of severe trauma and stress who have not come to terms with what they witnessed or heard within a few weeks often struggle with a lack of control over triggers, flashbacks, or intrusive thoughts. Learning and applying the techniques outlined in this book can help them regain that control—not only over their mental and physical experiences, but over their lives as a whole.

To ensure the text is as widely accessible as possible, it is intentionally written jargon- and psychobabble-free.

Another purpose of this book is to give *hope* to both survivors and practitioners. Stories abound from those working in this field where survivors have not only learned to manage life after trauma but have gone on to live fuller lives, thriving lives. This applies equally to victims of armed robbery, near-death experiences, rape and sexual assault, terrorist incidents, adult survivors of child abuse and neglect, natural disasters, sudden deaths, and road traffic incidents involving death and carnage.

Although this book takes a solution-focused approach, with many techniques drawn from either solution-focused or cognitive-behavioural therapies, practitioners from other therapeutic traditions can also incorporate these techniques into their practice.

Introduction

In the following pages, you will find over 130 tools and techniques that have helped tens of thousands of survivors of various types of severe trauma and stress. The emphasis is on simplicity and effectiveness, with a minimum of jargon as far as possible.

The book's contents are primarily directed at survivors, serving essentially as their personal guide. However, as I outline the various techniques, you will notice that I am addressing both survivors and practitioners.

If you are a worker/practitioner—counsellor, therapist, psychologist, psychiatrist, medical officer/doctor, welfare worker, helpline worker or experienced lay worker—you will find the contents of this handbook an invaluable addition to your "toolbox" when working with all kinds of survivors. Your fellow practitioners have been using and field-testing these tools and techniques for years. The evidence base for the solution-focused approach is now well established (see Appendix I).

In addition, the practice-based evidence continues to grow, and more importantly, the personal testimonies of survivors of death, carnage, or other traumatic events—who have regained control and gone on to live relatively trouble-free and fulfilling lives—continue to accumulate.

As practitioners, I believe we have both an ethical responsibility and a duty of care to undertake this important work, rather than simply medicating for symptom alleviation or providing "support". When workers avoid engaging in this work or rely on inappropriate treatments, the outcomes for the survivors can be unsatisfactory at best and tragic at worst. Stories of the latter are all too numerous to mention.

The pages ahead aim to equip workers not only with greater confidence but also the fullest range of tools and techniques to support them in delivering more effective treatment. If you need inspiration and encouragement right now, you may find it helpful to begin with Appendices A–G first before proceeding to the main sections of the book.

You may find yourself reading through the pages of this book on behalf of a friend or relative who is currently going through a difficult time. "Buddy-aid" can be powerful, and you might be surprised at just how helpful you can be.

You may have survived a recent (or not-so-recent) road traffic incident and still find yourself affected by certain thoughts, images, or avoidance reactions. This book is here to help you lay those thoughts, images, and feelings to rest. While memories of traumatic incidents stay with us (they do fade a little with time), the main objective of trauma recovery work is for survivors *to no longer be affected by trauma.* I will never forget all the awful things I experienced—both as a child and as an adult—but I have learned that I can live a full and productive life despite them. Unashamedly, I am now a "thriver".

Perhaps you witnessed someone die, be killed, or maimed right before your eyes. Maybe you have experienced much death and carnage. If so, you may find this book helpful. And if you are a survivor of a near-death ("near-miss") experience and often find yourself reflecting on what might have happened, this book is for you too. Whatever trauma you might have experienced, there is something here for you.

For some survivors, it will take courage and resolve to pick up this book and thumb through its pages to see what might be helpful for yourself or others. This does not mean you have "gone soft," or "weak," or somehow less of a person. In fact, often quite the opposite is the case. By following some—or many—of the suggestions in the sections that follow, you can become even stronger and more resilient than you already are. You, too, can look forward to living a fuller and more satisfying life.

A spin-off could also be that you find yourself in a better position to help others who may be in need. Where feelings of guilt, fear, shame, or anxiety may have been present, you can replace them with a renewed sense of direction and purpose in life.

You will notice that the text in this book is spaced more generously and set in a larger point size. This is to make this handbook even more user-friendly and accessible.

When trying out various tools and techniques within the six sections, if one does not work for you (or your client), it is not about "failure". It simply means that the tool or technique isn't the right fit at this point in time, and you may need to try another. This aligns well with a basic principle of the solution-focused approach: "going with what works".

How to Use
This Book

You will find that the tools and techniques in this book are organised into the following six sections:

1. Triggers
2. Flashbacks
3. Unwelcome thoughts
4. Dealing with 'the lows'
5. Disturbed sleep
6. Thriving/Living life to the full: increased meaning and purpose in life

For quick results, you may go directly to the section that best applies to your situation. Within each section, often the term "horses for courses" applies. Some survivors find one tool or technique particularly helpful, while others experiment with several before moving on. All the tools and techniques are available to try. It is often about finding "what works". The case studies will be helpful too.

The Term "Survivor"

Throughout the book, I have used the term "survivor". It simply refers to the fact that whatever traumatic event you have experienced or been a victim of, or that has befallen you, you have survived it.

Sometimes, survivor may carry a slightly different meaning to "survivor" within the Victim–Survivor–Thriver continuum, as outlined in Appendix D.

Deliberately, I have avoided using any other terms with negative connotations or could be disempowering in any way.

Acknowledgements

First, I would like to thank Steve de Shazer, the co-founder of Solution-Focused Brief Therapy, who inspired me to become involved in this specialist area of work after attending a 2-day workshop he presented in London in the early 1990s.

Second, I would like to thank Yvonne Dolan, a fellow survivor and thriver, who has devoted a big part of her life to working with survivors of severe trauma and stress. In the early days, Yvonne's help—through her workshops, her writing (N.B.: *Beyond Survival: Living Well is the Best Revenge*), and her personal words of encouragement—provided me with great impetus to get more involved in this important work. This was both for my work as a psychotherapist and a trainer.

I am grateful, as ever, to my wife, Lynn, who periodically has suggested I write this book due to "the need that is out there". She has been very understanding of my wish to "go away to the coast and write". She has worn well the mantle of "wordsmith's widow".

I am also grateful to Dr. Alasdair Macdonald for his encouragement and support with this project. This came first in the form of inspiring articles, suggestions of new avenues to explore, and in the form of useful books loaned. His permission to reproduce a short form evaluation list from his website (www.solutionsdoc.co.uk), thus sharing the evidence base for SFBT, was much appreciated (see Appendix I).

I would like to thank Prof. Harry Procter for casting his eye over later drafts of the manuscript and for making some useful suggestions regarding both the design and content of the first edition.

I am very grateful to my former secretaries, Joy Minnitt and Alison Wright, for all their diligent work on this project.

Finally, I would like to thank my many clients over the past 30 years who have applied the many techniques within the book to their lasting benefit. The results they achieved surprised them at the time. In the early days, I confess, I was surprised too!

About the Author

John Henden, BA (Hons) RMN Dip. Couns. (University of Bristol) MBACP FRSA, is an adult survivor of severe and enduring childhood abuse and neglect. He has had numerous traumatic experiences as an adult, including a near-drowning, three road traffic crashes, and a hold-up at knife-point in a mental hospital. These numerous experiences went unresolved and undeclared for many years; it is no surprise, therefore, that he experienced numerous bouts of "acute depression" for some considerable time. Through a combination of self-help and psychotherapy, not only could he declare himself a "survivor," but he has gone on to be a "thriver" (see Appendix D).

John has a background in psychology and is a solution-focused therapist, having specialised in severe trauma and stress recovery for over 30 years. In addition to being an author, he is a mental health consultant, visiting university lecturer, workshop presenter, broadcaster, and performance coach.

John is a regular presenter at European Brief Therapy Association conferences and is a founding member of SOLWorld. For the past 25 years, he has worked in over 25 countries across five continents.

He has worked in mental health, emotional well-being, welfare, and psychological support services for nearly 50 years, gaining both deep knowledge and a wide experience of "what works" when it comes to helping individuals get their lives back on track. Throughout his career, he has never lost sight of the potential in people to make the necessary changes to live useful and productive lives, despite earlier debilitating labels they may have been given. In addition to Solution-Focused Severe Trauma and Stress Recovery, John's other specialist interest subjects are Adult Survivors of Childhood Abuse and Neglect, Healthy Work–Life Balance, and Suicide Prevention.

With all the above, John feels more than a little qualified to write this book.

Contents

Dedication ix

Disclaimer...xi

The Book's Purpose xiii

Introduction xvii

How to Use This Book..xxi

The Term "Survivor" xxiii

Acknowledgements xxv

About the Author xxvii

Section 1   **Dealing with "Triggers"** 1

Section 2   **How to Deal with Flashbacks**................. 11

Section 3   **How to Deal with
               Unwelcome Thoughts** 25

Section 4   **Dealing with "The Lows"** 71

Section 5   **Dealing with Sleep Disturbance**............. 83

Section 6   **Living Life to the Full (or, as Full
               as Possible)** 105

Appendix A   **Reassuring Things for Survivors
               to Know** 151

Appendix B   **What Survivors Have Found to be Helpful in This Work** 153

Appendix C   **Helpful Questions and Statements from the Welfare Worker** 157

Appendix D   **The Three Stages: Victim–Survivor–Thriver (Living Life to the Full, or as Full as Possible)** 161

Appendix E   **The 5 o'clock Rule (for the First Sessions)** 167

Appendix F   **Blocks to Disclosing** 169

Appendix G   **How to Avoid Retraumatisation and Revictimisation** 173

Appendix H   **Benefits of Doing This Important Work** 175

Appendix I   **Two-Day Solution-Focused Workshops on Working with Severe Trauma and Stress** 179

Appendix J   **Supporting Research Evidence for Solution-Focused Brief Therapy** 185

Bibliography 207

Index 213

Section

Dealing with "Triggers"

1. **"That was then, this is NOW!"**
2. **"This is normal…"**
3. **"Breathe it away…"**
4. **Welcoming triggers through mindfulness**
5. **The 5-4-3-2-1 method**
6. **Name it – and identify the source**
7. **Use humour**

A trigger is something (e.g. a sight, sound, smell, taste, or bodily sensation) that sets off a reaction, taking you back to a particular event or situation. Triggers are highly unpredictable. Fighting, fearing, freezing, or fleeing from triggers *does not work* in the long term. It is better to *face* them and deal with them. So, instead of going for avoidance, go for acceptance. Dealing with them takes out their sting and enables us to remain in control. Also, it prevents the trigger from developing into a full-on "flashback" (see Section 2).

The strong suggestion in this manual is not to run from or try to avoid triggers, but to *welcome* them. This allows us to take control, practise the necessary techniques, and gain mastery over them. The result is often (surprise, surprise!) that the triggers occur less frequently, and when they do, they are dealt with easily and effectively. Welcoming them enables us to expose ourselves to events or situations in a way that is not harmful, and to live our lives to the full, regardless.

The Tools and Techniques

1. "That was then, this is NOW!"

This technique is very powerful for arresting a trigger in its tracks. It ensures that control remains with the survivor, not with the trigger, which could easily develop into a flashback.

The secret is to practise saying, **"That was then, this is** *NOW...!"* regularly, so that it can be used in an instant. It is important for welfare workers in this session to encourage survivors to slow down their pace of speech, lower their tone of voice, and say the sentence *forcefully*, with emphasis on the *"NOW…!"*

With this technique held in readiness, triggers—which are highly unpredictable—need not be feared; instead, they may be *welcomed*.

"Bring on the triggers!"

One survivor who had been traumatised over a number of years reported that on average, he encounters one trigger roughly every 2 weeks, but that this is not a problem now. By using this technique for just a few seconds on every occasion, he continues to live life to the full, regardless. He added that he now looks forward to the triggers occurring, so he can both practise and prove to himself that the technique works, *and* experience being in control.

"The smell of pork ribs"

A firefighter who responded to a house fire where several occupants had died after being badly burned, said that, as a result, he had avoided going to barbecues. He found the smell of cooking meat—especially where pork ribs were being served—just too much to bear. Clearly, he had been missing out on many potentially enjoyable family and other social gatherings for a few years.

Although he avoided barbecues he was invited to, he could not avoid the smell of his neighbours' barbecues wafting across his backyard whenever they chose to have one.

By learning and practising "That was then, this is *NOW*...!", and by accepting invitations to others' barbecues and holding one of his own, he proved that he had gained full control of his trigger.

2. "This is normal..."

Another way to gain mastery over a trigger is to train survivors to say quietly and firmly to themselves: "THIS IS NORMAL..." Instruct them that as soon as the trigger is observed, they should become consciously aware of it, see it for what it is, and say to themselves: "This is normal. These experiences occur from time to time. I am noticing them fully. And they will pass." In addition to being simple and easy to learn, this statement offers great reassurance.

"Gunfire — no problem"

A soldier who had returned from a 6-month tour of duty in an overseas territory happened to be walking his dog along a riverside path, well out in the country. Suddenly, he heard the sound of short bursts of machine gunfire from an army barracks in the distance. Naturally, thoughts of his tour of duty came rushing back, and he found himself in a difficult situation on one particular occasion. He was able to prevent this trigger from developing into a full-blown flashback by calmly and firmly saying out loud: "This is normal. I am bound to hear the sound of gunfire or other similar sounds from time to time, when I am out and about near military bases."

3. "Breathe it away"

This is another powerful technique for gaining control over triggers. Often, triggers can lead to the survivor taking a sharp in-breath. As described below, this technique enables survivors to maintain control by regulating their breathing. As a welfare worker/practitioner, you can provide the following instruction:

> When the trigger occurs, take control by first naming the experience (sight, sound, smell, taste, or bodily sensation) as a trigger. Then, slowly breathe out using your diaphragm (this means ensuring your stomach goes in on the out-breath and out on the in-breath). Often referred to as 7–11 breathing, this technique is simple. Breathe in gently and slowly through the nose for a count of 7, ensuring that your stomach expands on the in-breath. Then, breathe out through the mouth for a count of 11. Practise this for a couple of minutes, six or seven times a week, over a period of 6–8 weeks. This ensures it is

bedded in fully as a technique for you to use at any time. It is worth practising this type of breathing even under normal circumstances, when no triggers are present. Not only will you be prepared when a trigger occurs, but you will also generally feel better, as it is effective for several reasons. Firstly, toxins from the depth of the lungs are expelled during the out-breath. Secondly, the internal organs are massaged by this type of (correct) breathing. Thirdly, because we feel better physically, we also feel more relaxed mentally.

This type of breathing is widely recommended for people to regain control for themselves when they are feeling out of control. Also, those who experience panic attacks find this technique highly beneficial.

"Breathing away loud bangs"

A woman who had been within 200 yards of a terrorist bomb blast that killed and injured dozens was deeply affected by any loud crash or bang she heard. Most often, the sounds came from dustbins being dropped, objects being thrown into metal skips, or up-and-over garage doors slamming.

With regular practice, she learned to instantly shift from a sharp in-take of breath to a slow out-breath, and then followed by the 7–11 breathing routine described above.

4. Welcoming triggers through mindfulness

This aligns well with the idea of replacing avoidance with acceptance, as outlined in the introduction to this section.

The technique powerfully counters the "fight or flight" response by disarming it. Here's how it works:

At the first whiff of a trigger, say "Ah. I recognise you!", "Welcome!", or something similar. This response is the complete opposite of trying to run from it or pushing it down or away. Simply acknowledge the trigger. Pause for a moment, then breathe gently for five times. It may help if you put a hand on your stomach to slow things down. Be aware of your breathing. Now, let the thought come. Do not develop it, simply let it be. What would help *at this moment?*

You will know. Stay with it. Now continue with gentle breathing, being in the moment. You may now choose to use techniques 1, 2, or 3, or the mindfulness technique alone may be sufficient.

5. The 5-4-3-2-1 method

The procedure outlined below is very useful for dealing with triggers, helping to pull survivors back to the here and now. (It is also effective for inducing sleep if awakened at night by internal or external events—see Section 4.)

The steps are as follows:

Open your eyes.
Notice five things you can see.

Close your eyes.
Notice five things you can hear.
Notice five things you feel in your body (e.g. warmth, pillows, etc.—focus on physical sensations, not emotions).

Open your eyes.
Notice four things you can see.

Close your eyes.
Notice four things you can hear.
Notice four things you feel in your body.

Open your eyes.
Notice three things you can see.

Close your eyes.
Notice three things you can hear.
Notice three things you feel in your body.

Open your eyes.
Notice two things you can see.

Close your eyes.
Notice two things you can hear.
Notice two things you feel in your body.

Open your eyes.
Notice one thing you can see.

Close your eyes.
Notice one thing you can hear.
Notice one thing you feel in your body.

Repeat if necessary to extinguish the trigger more firmly.

After practising the exercise four or five times, it will become easier, and the calming effect will be greater.

6. Name it – and identify the source

This technique is a variation on the theme of the previous five techniques.

As soon as the trigger is identified, *name it* (a person, word, smell, taste, sound, place, behaviour facial expression, etc.), and then *identify the source* of the trigger reaction—a specific event.

This process often greatly reduces the trigger's impact.

"The scary member of the interview panel"

A woman applying for a job was called into the interview room and met by a panel of four interviewers. Immediately, she noticed that one of them had "scary eyes."

Naming "scary eyes" was the first step; the second was: "looks a bit like how my mother used to look at me when she was being emotionally abusive."

7. Use humour

On noticing the trigger, quickly divert to a humorous response. This is a fast way to diffuse the stress response, thus avoiding a flashback.

Example

A man in his forties, noticing someone in a meeting who resembled an abusive teacher from schooldays, said quietly to himself: "There's 'an Old Wrighty lookalike'. I bet he'll have a high-pitched squeaky voice when he speaks!"

How to Deal with Flashbacks

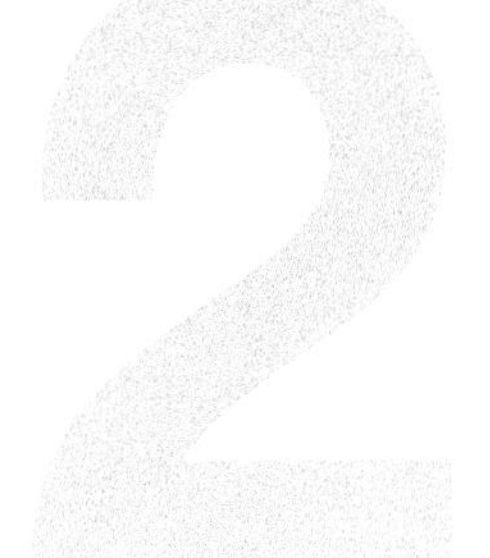

1. "Shrinking" (or the "reversing") technique
2. Dual awareness
3. The rewind technique
4. Confronting the flashbacks head-on
5. Eye movement desensitisation and reprocessing (EMDR)
6. Voluntarily, bring on a pleasant flashback

Definition of a flashback: "a recurrence of a memory, feeling or perceptual experience from the past" (DSM-V, 2013).

Flashbacks, which are normal, may be triggered by sights, sounds, smells, or feelings. The aim is to disrupt these triggers in their tracks by using the techniques in

Section 1 to avoid a resulting flashback. Using techniques for flashbacks can be described as a "second line of defence". Unless we deal with them effectively as they arise, flashbacks can cause us to feel trapped, powerless, and/or out of control. We may feel at the mercy of our experiences. *This need not happen*, as will be seen in the following pages.

The tools and techniques for dealing with them are easy to learn and apply.

In addition to negative flashbacks, there can be positive ones too, which can bring about pleasant experiences. We can induce these voluntarily and consciously to demonstrate to ourselves that not only can we be in control, but that pleasant flashbacks are possible.

We do this by recalling past triggers in the form of a pleasant sight, sound, touch, taste, or smell. A case example of this is provided below.

There follows a helpful selection of techniques to help manage flashbacks of unpleasant experiences. What is of fundamental importance is to arrest the flashback in its tracks to minimise its impact.

The Tools and Techniques

1. "Shrinking" (or the "reversing") technique

The "shrinking" technique is a powerful and effective way for tackling flashbacks, particularly when the experience involves approaching missiles of any kind. It has been used most effectively with military personnel who have faced such battlefield situations, as well as with vehicle drivers involved in serious road traffic incidents where debris from other vehicles or entire vehicles have come towards them at speed.

The effectiveness of this technique, like so many others, lies in regaining power and control. Instead of the distressing psychological and physical sequence of events that might be experienced, survivors take control and "dispose" of the incoming missile in a novel, safe, and more comfortable way. Over time, this reduces the severity of the flashback's effects until it no longer holds power at all.

This is easy for practitioners to teach and easy for survivors to learn on their own.

Instructions for the technique are as follows:

What I invite you to do is to visualise the missile coming towards you. As it approaches, allow yourself to get a good look at it… At the moment just before impact, in your mind's eye… stop the missile in its tracks… Now, send it back in a different direction towards the distant *horizon*. As it travels along this new path, *change its colour to any colour* you choose… As it travels further away, notice how much *smaller* it gets… until it becomes a mere speck on the horizon. And if you keep watching, you will notice that you can no longer see it at all.

It is important to practise this at least three times a week for around 6 weeks. If, during some weeks, you only manage two practice sessions instead of three, that is okay. As you practise, notice the ways in which you find it helpful or useful.

After practising this technique on a number of occasions, some survivors rename it as the "reversing" technique.

"The car wreckage missile — sorted"

An experienced driver of 40-tonne, six-axle lorries was involved in a fatal road crash in which three passengers, travelling in two separate vehicles, were killed.

A car, which had been overtaking him, crashed head-on with an oncoming lorry about 40 yards ahead. The estimated impact speed was between 100 and 110 mph. A front wheel of the overtaking car, with attached steering rods, flew through the air at great speed towards the driver's windscreen, hitting it with a giant "thwack!", before bouncing off and away. He knew he would have been killed if the windscreen had been smashed. For this driver, triggers into flashbacks of this event were seeing windscreens of passing lorries, department store windows bulging slightly as doors opened and closed, traffic passing, or even just the wind.

Initially, he tried dealing with the triggers by using the "That was then, this is *NOW*…!" technique. However, before he had mastered this technique, he noticed that the full flashback would occur rapidly. To manage this, he practised the "shrinking" technique at a regular time each day for a few weeks. This enabled him to have control over both the trigger and the full flashback to the crash should it occur again. He was able to gain control over it by changing them in the way outlined above. As a result, the flashbacks became less severe and occurred less frequently. They stopped altogether after about 4–5 months.

2. Dual awareness[a]

This powerful technique comes with the following instructions. When learning it, make sure to say the words slowly, deliberately, and with a strong voice:

"It seems we have got two things going on here."

Right now, I am feeling (isolated/lonely/fearful/etc.[a]) and I am sensing in my body… (three or so physical sensations: heart racing, perspiring, tremulousness, etc.[a])

---

[a] Adapted from a protocol drawn up by Rothschild (2000). *Note*: Delete the words that do not apply to you; adding others, as appropriate. If you are a practitioner, it is helpful to have this dual awareness technique on a database for you to adapt to each client's unique situation.

These are real sensations—that's what I am experiencing right now—because I am remembering the traumatic event/explosion/incident/abuse/hold-up/assault/robbery/accident/etc.[a]

However, at the same time, I am looking around where I am now here (the place/room[a] where I am now) and:

I can see five things…   (name them)
I can hear five things…   (name them)
I can sense the following five things…   (name them)

And so, I know the traumatic event/explosion/incident/abuse/hold-up/assault/robbery/accident/etc.[a] is not happening now or anymore.

"Fireworks: where did they come from!"

A veteran of the first Gulf War was walking through his local park one summer evening, as a "Prom in the Park" event was drawing to a close. A few minutes later, all hell seemed to break loose for him as the firework display began with a flash and a bang.

Immediately, he had the beginnings of a full-blown flashback of being in Saudi Arabia, where an incoming Iraqi Scud missile exploded into a hangar just a few dozen yards away from him.

He applied the **dual awareness technique**, as follows:

"It seems I have two things going on here. **Right now,** I am feeling terrified and sensing, in my body, a racing heart, eyes wide and alert, a tightening in my stomach, and sweaty hands. I want to run and take cover.

These are real sensations—this is what I am experiencing right now—because I am remembering the Scud missile attack from all those years ago.

However, at the same time, I am looking around where I am now, here in the park, and I can see five things:

— The orchestra playing;
— The smiling, delighted faces of the audience;
— The beautiful colours of the fireworks;
— The moon, partially covered by clouds;
— The grass I see everywhere looked quite a deep dark green.

I can hear five things:

— The whoosh of the rockets as they rush heavenwards;
— The pleasant sound of violins;
— The chatter of groups of friends watching;

— The clinking of bottles and wine glasses;
— The distant hum of the evening traffic.

I can sense the following five things:

— The smell of the firework smoke;
— The gentle breeze on the side of my face;
— My shoes against the soft turf of the park;
— The sulphurous taste of the smoke;
— My left thumb struggling to get out through the hole in my glove!

And so I know, the Scud attack in Saudi Arabia is not happening now or anymore."

Once the exercise was completed, the war veteran wandered on, taking in the atmosphere of both the concert and the fireworks, having regained his composure and control.

3. The rewind technique[b]

The rewind technique should be learned and practised under the guidance of an experienced practitioner and

---

[b]This technique was developed by Richard Bandler of the NLP fame. He, in turn, got it from Milton Erickson, who invited clients to look at themselves inside a crystal ball. Griffin & Tyrrell (2004) have developed the idea into an even more powerful form.

works in about 90% of cases. It is carried out in a state of deep relaxation or trance.

Once relaxed, clients are asked to recall or imagine a place where they feel totally safe and at ease. This is their special place. Their relaxed state is then deepened. Next, they are asked to imagine that within their special place, they have a TV set and a DVD player with a remote-control facility. This time, they are asked to imagine themselves floating outside of their body, and witness themselves watching the traumatic event on TV. (This method is one way to create a significant emotional distance.) Then, they are asked to rewind the trauma as if it were happening in real life. Next, they relive it as if in real life—this creates what is called "kinaesthetic visualisation". The film begins at a point before the trauma occurred—a point of safety— and ends at a point at where the trauma is over and they feel safe again. After this, they float back into their body and imagine pressing the DVD rewind button on the remote control, watching themselves quickly going backward through the trauma, from safe point to safe point. Then, they watch the same images again, but going forward very quickly, as if pressing the fast-forward button.

All this is repeated back and forth, at a pace dictated by the individual concerned and as many times as needed, until the scenes no longer evoke any emotion. They are asked to go forward and backward about four times, which seems, in most cases, to be sufficient in dealing with the traumatic memory.

If the goal is to instill confidence to face the feared circumstance in the future—for instance, driving a car or using a lift—they are asked to imagine a scenario in which they are doing so while feeling confident and relaxed. Once accomplished, clients are brought out of the trance, marking the completion of the rewind technique.

Besides being safe, quick, painless, and side-effect free, this technique has the advantage of being non-voyeuristic. Intimate details do not have to be voiced. It is the client who watches the "film", not the welfare worker.

4. Confronting the flashbacks head-on

By this time, if you have not succeeded in identifying and dealing with the trigger, say the following to yourself:

"Okay, so this is a flashback. But, I know deep down that the worst is over because the feelings and sensations I am having belong to the past."

"I am here now, in the present, so let's get the control back!"

Four simple steps to do this are as follows:

1. Pinch yourself or press one foot on top of the other.

2. Breathe normally, overemphasising both the out-breaths and in-breaths. Breathe on the out-breath to the count of 11 and on each in-breath to the count of 7. (Make sure to use your diaphragm when breathing, as described above under "Breathe it away").

3. Re-establish yourself in the present by using the five senses:
    i. I can see five things…
    ii. I can hear five things…
    iii. I can feel five things…
    iv. I can taste, smell, or sense five things…

4. Notice the particular ways in which you are regaining control.

5. Voluntarily, bring on a pleasant flashback

Perhaps it can be said that each of us have a wonderful collection of fond and happy memories from the past. Whether this be from early childhood, our teenage years, or more recent times. This is a good opportunity to prove you can be in control at will. Bring on one of these pleasant flashbacks through a particular sight, memory, smell, taste, or sensation. By doing this for ourselves, we become better able to describe its benefits and more capable and effective to teach it to others.

"The sweet perfume of roses"

An adult survivor of severe and enduring multiple child abuse recalled a regular summer holiday spent at a small guest house in a coastal resort. Although he was abused by both parents—and they also emotionally abuse each other—this annual trip was a relatively "happy" window in each unhappy year.

It so happened that the main passion of the guest house proprietor was cultivating rare varieties of garden roses. The survivor, back then a young boy, seldom missed the daily opportunity to take a deep, nose-full of scent from vividly coloured roses in the garden. Over the years, he continued to indulge in this habit, sniffing garden roses whenever the opportunity presented itself.

He enabled the trigger (the roses' scent) to develop into a full-blown flashback to the many happy holidays of his childhood by the sea.

6. Eye movement desensitisation and reprocessing (EMDR)[c]

This form of treatment has helped hundreds of thousands of people worldwide who have suffered from a wide range of traumatic events.

---

[c]Some warnings about EMDR: With some individuals, there is a risk of dizziness with this technique. So, those who easily get dizzy are not advised to do this. Often,

EMDR involves stimulating eye movement in a way that activates the brain's information-processing systems. Amazingly, negative internal messages are squashed instantly as the person's eyes flicker back and forth, side to side, while focusing on the painful memory.

The instructions for survivors are as follows:

1. I want you to sit comfortably in front of me.
2. Now, for about a minute, shift your eyes rapidly from side to side while focusing on the incident. To help keep your eyes on track, use your closed fist with two fingers up in a V sign, held about a foot in front of you, and move it side to side.
3. Continue the pendulum action with your hand for the full minute, focusing fully on the incident.
4. Towards the end of the minute, mentally picture the worst part of the incident. Now, keep that image in focus while continuing to shift your eyes in this lateral position.
5. With the image clearly in focus and eyes shifting back and forth, feel your entire body engulfed in panic.

this technique can be very effective in removing symptoms in the short term, but they can resurface again unexpectedly later on. You will then need to repeat the exercise. Like all the tools and techniques within this book, this is another technique for your toolbox, for you to try out.

6. Take full account of how your discomfort is spreading from top to bottom and allow it to flow freely without resisting.
7. Now, stop the anxiety abruptly by taking a deep breath using your diaphragm.
8. Stop the mental image.
9. Refocus on the left-to-right movement of your two fingers, concentrating on them fully.
10. You will notice, hypnotically, that you begin to feel less anxiety and become more entranced as your eyes follow your two fingers shifting back and forth.
11. Focus on the left and right movement of your two fingers, concentrating on them fully.

Section

How to Deal with Unwelcome Thoughts

1. The "Stop!" technique and Replaying the DVD later
2. Tackle the guilt trip
3. "Tell it—don't bottle it"
4. "Get in some 'degrimming' or black humour"
5. The letter from the future
6. Changing the mindset
7. How to beat the "If only..." monster on your shoulder
8. Write, read, and burn
9. "Park it... and move on..."
10. "Let it go... Let it go... Let it go..."
11. Fast-forwarding the live stream of your life
12. Ways to deal with anger build-ups

13.   **Change your mental attitude towards unwelcome thoughts**

14.   **Visualisation**

15.   **The solution-focused feelings tank**

Intrusive (or unwelcome or unwanted) thoughts are common to people. These are thoughts that find their way, often repeatedly, into our everyday thinking. They may develop into the "flashbacks" previously mentioned, or can be simply irritating and annoying interruptions to whatever we are doing at the time. They can prevent us from living happy and fulfilled lives. To stop them from causing us emotional or psychological distress, we must deal with them effectively.

The following are many useful tools and techniques that can help survivors combat these unwanted thoughts. By practising them, they will be able to continue whatever activity they are involved in with little to no disturbance.

1. The "Stop!" technique and Replaying the DVD later

This technique is highly effective for dealing with regularly occurring intrusive thoughts.

Intrusive thoughts are unpredictable and can occur any time during waking hours—from the very moment you wake up until the last moment before you sleep at night.

The "Stop!" technique addresses the issues of both "control" and "boundarying", as to start with, there are no boundaries to the experiences.

First, the survivor needs to make a decision to take control. This is done by wearing a rubber band on a wrist of their choice. The rubber band should be neither too tight nor too loose, so it can be worn comfortably without causing a red mark. A very thin band is ideal, as it delivers a more painful sting when snapped against the wrist.

Once applied to the wrist, the survivor is invited to practise snapping the rubber band. (It is more effective if the practitioner demonstrates it first, modelling the experience of both the snapping and the pain.)

The instructions are as follows:

1. As soon as the intrusive thought occurs, reach for the rubber band and snap it against your wrist while firmly saying, "Stop!".

2. As you say "Stop!", think to yourself: "I will give this incident some thinking time later".

3. Carry on with whatever you were doing or thinking about before the intrusive thought occurred.

4. Continue using the "Stop!" technique throughout the day, every time an intrusive thought occurs.

5. In the early evening (at least 2 hours before bedtime), spend 20–30 minutes replaying the incident, as if

you were watching it all on a DVD. Begin at a point where all was safe, peaceful, and quiet before the incident. Then, go through each aspect of the incident to its end, and then to the point where safety, peace, and quiet are restored.

6. Repeat this process every day for as long as necessary.

(NB: It is important to "Replay the DVD" at least 2 hours before retiring to bed, so the person can be involved in other thoughts and activities before bedtime. This minimises the risk of the incident's vivid details being worked out in dreams or nightmares.)

There have been some amazing results achieved with this twin technique. Intrusive thoughts have been reduced from around 80–90 per day to just 5–6 per week within approximately 5 weeks.

At first, survivors have been keen to spend a full 20–30 minutes to the "replay" stage. However, over time, they find they need less time, and the repetition becomes boring—eventually, they stop altogether. This is perfectly fine, as it demonstrates that the technique has served its purpose.

While some reddening of the wrists may occur in the early days of using "Stop!", the need to use it lessens. This is because the brain learns it is being "punished" when thinking about the incident outside the time boundary in the early evening.

"The robbery: conquering the aftermath"

A female university student, who was earning extra cash by working evening shifts at her local "off licence", was the victim of an armed robbery while cashing up at 10:00 pm. Two balaclava-clad men rushed in, pointed a handgun at her, and demanded the day's takings along with several hundred cigarettes. For a couple of weeks afterward, she experienced recurrent nightmares and was having up to 80 intrusive thoughts per day—particularly the men's wild-looking eyes and the shiny parts of their handgun.

After using the "Stop!" technique for 1 week, the intrusive thoughts had reduced to 4–5 per day, and the nightmares had all stopped.

With the "replaying of the DVD" part of this technique, more power can be provided by incorporating "the paper strips method". The instructions for this are as follows:

1. Fold five A4-sized sheets of white paper in half horizontally.
2. Press hard along the crease with your thumbnail, then tear each sheet in half. This will give you two sets of five sheets (now A5-sized).

3. Fold each A5 sheet in half again horizontally.

4. Repeat the tearing process along the new crease.

5. Continue folding and tearing until you have 40 (5 × 8) strips of paper.

6. Fold two sheets of coloured A4-sized paper horizontally, as instructed above.

7. Continue folding and tearing until the two coloured sheets produce 16 strips.

8. Now, referring to step 5, replay the incident— beginning with what you were doing before it began.

9. With each part of the story, place one white strip on the table.

10. Place a coloured strip each time you remember something you did well—such as a personal quality, strength, or characteristic that you brought into play, or something you were pleased about.

11. Continue this process through the entire incident, up to the point when equilibrium was restored or a point of safety was reached.

12. You should end up with a giant, multi-layered "paper strip sandwich" of both white and coloured paper strips. Usually, survivors end up with a white-to-coloured strip ratio of about 4:1.

There is a three-fold purpose in adding "the paper strips method" to this technique:

A. It reduces the risk of retraumatisation, as strengths, qualities, and other positive points punctuate the story.
B. It empowers the survivor, as they take more control over their story while "replaying the DVD" to themselves.
C. It speeds up the time when boredom kicks in. The brain will eventually become fed up with repeating the same exercise day after day and will want to be occupied with something else more interesting.

The "Stop!" technique and replaying the DVD later, along with the paper strips, has been highly effective in reducing intrusive or unwelcome thoughts for many people.

It is best illustrated by the following example.

A lorry driver was travelling along a curved section of a single carriageway bypass when he noticed a motorcyclist approaching him. Being a motorcyclist himself, he thought the rider was going too fast for the bend and was poorly positioned on his side of the road.

The lorry driver slowed to about 40 mph, hoping the motorcyclist would do the same. Within seconds, he saw the motorcyclist's terrified expression as he hit the front of the cab at an impact speed of over 90 mph. For about a week after the incident, the driver was having 70–80 flashbacks per day. Adding the paper strips method to replaying the DVD, the exercise went as follows:

— "There I was, driving along the open road at a steady 50 mph.

— lays down one white strip (WS)

— The sun was shining and there were a few puffy white clouds in the sky.

— WS

— I was listening to a play on Radio 4 and, since it was mid-afternoon, there was not much traffic around.

— WS

— I could see a motorcyclist about 200 yards away, coming towards me. He seemed to be going too fast for the curve.

— WS

— I slowed down to about 40 mph as he continued approaching at speed.

— lays down green strip (GS)

— He was still coming fast into the curve, and both his road positioning and "lean" were all wrong.

— WS

— He was coming straight towards my cab, so I braked sharply and safely, slowing down quickly.

— GS

— I saw his terrified expression, and he seemed to be mouthing the words, "Oh God!"

— WS

— There was a terrific bang and a jolt to my cab. I travelled a bit further, scraping wreckage until I brought my vehicle to a halt.

— WS

— I put the lorry into gear, applied the handbrake, turned off the ignition, picked up my mobile phone, and stepped down from the cab.

— GS

— I took a quick glance at the mangled bike wreckage and the dead rider. He was beyond help.

— WS

— I phoned 999 and gave them an accurate location of the incident.

— GS

— Other vehicles had slowed down and stopped.

— WS

— There was already a driver directing traffic.

— WS

— I informed the other drivers and passengers who were approaching to stay away from the front of the lorry for their own safety. There was nothing to be done for the rider, and, that the emergency services were already on their way.

— GS

— Another two drivers agreed to direct traffic.

— WS

— I returned to my cab to call my transport manager and inform him of the incident.

— GS

— I switched the radio to a music channel to calm my nerves while waiting for the emergency services to arrive.

— GS

— The police arrived first.

— WS

— I got down from the cab and locked it behind me, in accordance with my driving rules.

— GS

— I sat in the police car and gave a statement.

— WS

— I noticed the ambulance arrive, and they removed the body.

— WS

— As the policeman was finishing his interview, I heard a fire and rescue tender arrive, just as the breakdown vehicle joined the scene.

— WS

— I returned to the cab to remove all personal items and my company documents that might have been under the dashboard.

— GS

— I had a lift home in the police patrol car.

— WS

— On the way, he said his colleague would be at the scene for some time, measuring skid marks on the road, etc.

— WS

— On the way, the policeman chatted reassuringly. He was a kind bloke and gave me a cup of hot, sweet tea from his own flask.

— GS

— He told me that he sees too many motorcycle fatalities in the course of his work.

— WS

— Once home, I had a hot bath, chucked in loads of bath salts, and lay there for about an hour and a half.

— GS

— I dressed and went downstairs to the kitchen, where I made myself a large mug of cocoa. All I could eat was a bowl of soup and some dry bread.

— GS

— I sat in my lounge, tried to watch TV before going to bed.

— WS"

2. Tackle the guilt trip

Two common unwelcome thoughts among many survivors of severe trauma are guilt and self-blame. Questions that keep intruding into the waking mind include:

"I feel so guilty because I survived and he died."

"Things went wrong and I am to blame."

"I feel so bad about it and it's all my fault!"

"My concentration dipped only for a few seconds. If only I had… it wouldn't have happened!"

When disturbing things like this happens to us, it is quite normal to have these intrusive thoughts of guilt or self-blame. It is often referred to as "survivor guilt".

There are two ways to deal with these feelings.

(a) *"It was not your fault"*

First, tell yourself it was *not your fault* or you are not to blame. In most situations, even though we may feel guilty, looking at the hard facts helps us discover that we are not to blame—that it was in no way our fault. Give the incident/situation a reality check.

"It was my fault the baby was killed"

A 19-year-old woman in a war zone was held captive in some farm buildings by about a dozen occupying troops. Among the 25 fellow captives was a mother carrying a 6-month-old baby. The baby was crying from hunger, so after dark, the teenager crept into an enclosure of dairy cows and milked one of them so the baby could be fed. When she returned, she was discovered by two of her captors, who promptly killed the baby as a punishment for the theft of the milk. For over 40 years, she told no one, carrying an enormous burden of guilt over the baby's death. It was not surprising that during that time, she suffered from anxiety, depression, and sleep disturbances.

Her therapist helped her look at the facts:

— She felt normal human compassion towards both the mother and her hungry baby.
— It was an act of human kindness to look for food to ease the baby's obvious distress.
— She ventured bravely into the night to milk one of the cows.
— The two occupying troops should take full responsibility for their cruel actions; she was not to blame.
— It was the troops who made the decision to kill the baby—not the young woman.

— No one can ask more of us than to do our best in whatever circumstances we find ourselves.

A final question that proved very helpful was this: "What skills, qualities, and resources did you bring to the fore to get through that ordeal—both at the time and over the ensuing months, until the end of the war?"

Over the final three sessions, the weight of guilt began to lift, and she felt much freer. In the last session, she shared her resolve to fulfil a lifelong dream of working with brain-injured children.

(b) *"You are not wholly to blame"*

In some situations, or in certain incidents, after taking a long, hard look at the facts, we may discover that we were to blame to some extent. The question to ask is this: *"Were you 100% to blame?"* In every case, you will find that the answer is "No". There is always someone else to share it.

This is illustrated best by the following example.

"I should have saved my son from suicide"

A divorced man in his fifties had three grown-up children. His son, the middle child, was living alone in a bedsitting room. He had experienced depressive episodes for a number of years and had sought help from his general practitioner (GP) on several occasions. Each time, he was prescribed with pills. About 6 months earlier, he spent around a month in a local psychiatric inpatient facility but discharged himself, saying, "… they just gave me more pills and observed me. The staff, apart from telling me where to go and what to do, didn't really seem to want to talk to me".

Over one long weekend, the man's son took his life by swallowing all his prescribed medication.

With the help of his counsellor, the father, who felt he was totally responsible for his son's death ("If I had been a better father…", "I should have gone round to see him more often…", "I could have paid for some decent counselling for him …, etc.), could appreciate that others shared the blame. With the counsellor's help, he came up with the following individuals and their approximate percentages of the total blame:

The GP, for prescribing pills only and not referring him to a reputable counsellor: 30%

The psychiatrist, who carried medical responsibility for his son's treatment in the hospital: 30%

The nursing staff in the unit, who seemed to want minimal interactions only with inpatients: 20%

His son, for not pressing his case for better help: 10%

Politicians, for underfunding mental health services: 20%

Manufacturers of psychiatric drugs, who convince doctors that their products are treatment rather than (in reality) simply symptom-alleviation: 20%

The community care worker, who was supposed to call round to the bedsit to see him following his discharge from the inpatient unit: 15%

Total for "others": 145%!

This often happens, where the total of the others' percentages exceeds 100%. However, the total can only be 100%, *including* the father's percentage. So, pressing him to take a share of this 100% helps him accept a realistic percentage of his part in the incident.

He believed he should carry approximately 20% of the blame. Once he had accepted his share, he was then helped in dealing with and coming to terms with that 20%. Subsequently, he resolved to join a support group for those bereaved by suicide, as a way of "paying back".

3. "Tell it—don't bottle it"

Bottling things up, suppressing them, or pushing them down has never done anyone any good. It may help us forget about things in the short term, but it is *not good for our health.*

If we push things down for any length of time, they will bubble up during the day when we least expect it, or surface at night in the form of vivid dreams and/or nightmares. Worse: they could come out in some form of psychosomatic problem or physical illness. As the saying goes, "What's pushed down, must come up later."

We need to express it safely, in some way or another. This may be done either by the spoken word, "writing, reading, and burning" or high-energy physical exercise (see both in Sections 4 and 6.)

Here are two helpful guiding statements:

- "It's good to talk."
- "A problem shared is a problem halved."

Be careful who you tell

Some people may struggle to cope with what they hear—especially if it is shocking, tragic, or both—and may protect themselves by simply not believing. Others may simply not understand at all. Some will glaze over while being told, while others may show little to no understanding or empathy. There are also those who cannot keep confidences and will be bursting to share what they have been told with others.

Finding the right person with whom you can share, in complete confidence, what has happened to you is both rewarding and liberating.

4. "Get in some 'degrimming' or black humour"

The ability to use humour or to "de-grim" situations with some quip or another is a quality that enables people to overcome even the most horrendous situations. There are countless examples of how this has been helpful across many situations and various traumatic events. Black humour has been used to good effect both during an incident and afterwards. It helps to lighten an otherwise grim situation, allowing us to deal with it on the spot and to "put it away" more safely in our memory—until such a time when it can be dealt with more effectively, if necessary.

Examples

1. Firefighters who responded to a fatal car crash: "One thing's for certain—she won't do that again!"
2. Ambulance staff at a failed suicide attempt from a bridge: "As he jumped, he didn't expect his overcoat to balloon out like a parachute!"
3. During an earthquake, a man who ran out of a collapsing building just in time: "I would have found myself at the Pearly Gates, sooner than I expected!"

5. The letter from the future[a]

This letter is to be written and not posted:

> Pick a time in the future—5, 10, 15, 20 years from now, or any number of years—longer or shorter—that is meaningful to you. Date the top of the letter with this imaginary future date. Now, imagine that all those intervening years have passed and you are writing to a friend (pick someone you know and like in the present time). Use the friend's name: "Dear (friend's name)". Or, if you prefer, pick another supportive person to whom you can comfortably imagine writing.

The purpose of dating the letter and writing it to someone you know, in reality, is to strengthen its psychological realism for you, both on a conscious and unconscious level. Imagine that in this future, you have resolved whatever problems that are troubling you at the present time. Describe what helped you resolve those problems. At the time of writing the letter, you are living a wonderful, joyous, healthy, and satisfying life. Describe how you spend your time, where you live, your relationships, your beliefs, and your reflections on the past and future.

---

[a] With full acknowledgement to Milton Erickson for the original version and to Yvonne Dolan for a later amended version.

How to use the letter from the future[b]

Now that you have completed the letter, what did you learn? What did you include in the letter that is not yet happening in your life? What would be the smallest[c] step in your actual behaviour or reactions that you could take towards making one of those things begin to happen? When do you want to try taking that step?

What difference would that small step make if it continued over time? Are other small steps needed now? What would be the next smallest one? What result(s) do you expect from each of the steps you can identify? When do you want to start? If you don't want to start, is it the wrong goal? If you do want to start but feel stuck, are there any advantages to not starting? If so, is there a way to preserve some of the advantages of not starting (such as

---

[b] With full acknowledgement to Yvonne Dolan.

[c] Sometimes people ask, "Why imagine the smallest sign, why not big, glorious signs?" The aim here is to make whatever changes you desire become unintimidating, to scale them down to a level that is comfortably achievable for you, so that your goal is reachable. It is not that people fail to make changes because they are lazy. What passes for laziness is usually fear, demoralisation, or despair. The smallness of these signs is intended to overcome fear and demoralisation, and to allow you to complete your own version of the Chinese proverb, "A journey of a thousand miles begins with a single step", one small achievable step at a time. If the steps you identify seem too small, simply make them slightly larger, taking care to make them no larger than is "do-able" in the next day or two. Then proceed. Remember, if the process stalls, or if you become overwhelmed or stuck, check to see if the goal is truly what you want, and if so, ask yourself if the step needs to be made smaller. Keep making it smaller until it is one you can do. Do not give up; you deserve the life you want.

extra time) without you remaining stuck? What might be the consequences (how will you feel in 5, 10, 15, 20 years) if you do not start?

The purpose of these questions is to identify your motivation. If you still want to start, do not be discouraged by the smallness of the steps. If you need inspiration for the power of small steps, go and interview a successful quilt maker, a writer, or a tile layer—or anyone whose work progresses gradually, piece by piece. In fact, what work does not progress gradually? You are your own greatest project!

6. Changing the mindset

This is a useful technique for survivors who have a fixed belief about a situation.

Before changing that (fixed) mindset, it is important to "loosen the negative thinking around the edges". This means sowing seeds of doubt about its validity; highlighting strengths, abilities, and resources within—and, if possible, flagging how some of these were already used in the situation. Also, questions, such as "What would you do more of or do differently next time, should a similar incident occur?" and "What might be the smallest, positive thing you have taken away from the incident?" may be helpful.

Once the edges of the negative thinking have been loosened sufficiently, the following types of statements can be made, as appropriate:

1. "You did the best you could under the circumstances."
2. "You were simply doing your job."
3. "You had to think and act quickly. Sometimes, in situations like this, mistakes are made."
4. "It was either you or them. What other choices did you have?"
5. "Sometimes on life's journey, shocking, distressing, frightening, or upsetting things like this happen to us. In what ways do you think this experience has made you a stronger person?"
6. "It seems you were in the right place at the right time."
7. "It seems you were in the wrong place at the right time."
8. "Sometimes in life, we do something terrible. However, rather than beating ourselves up about it, we can try to forgive ourselves. We may ask for God's forgiveness too."
9. "With some things that happen, for which we feel responsible, we can pay back in some way by doing good deeds for others. What might you do if you were so inclined?"

10. "You can either look at your injuries as 'the end of the world', or you can decide how you can live life to the full despite them."

11. "What would you say you have learned as a result of this experience?"

12. You may add your own, which can be statements, questions, or a combination of both.

7. How to beat the "If only..." monster on your shoulder

"**If only**…" can be a handicapping, recurrent thought, as it has the powerful effect of keeping us stuck in the present.

Severe trauma and stress survivors have found this technique both highly effective and fun to do.

The technique for dealing with it is an adaptation of what was used by Jacob (2001) when working with eating distress. With this technique, survivors are encouraged to "externalise the problem" by visualising it as sitting on their shoulder, such that it can be seen as an object in its own right rather than as an internal part of themselves.

Once it is sitting on your shoulder, not only can you get a good look at its entirety, you can also get into direct and assertive conversation with it. The objective of these conversations is to beat it, outsmart it, defeat it, or put it on the back foot. Most survivors prefer the phrase "beat it" because of its triple meaning: "successfully argue against it", "beat it physically", and "persuade it to beat it (leave altogether)."

"If only…", if allowed to persist, is very controlling and disempowering. Survivors must regain both power and control, and this technique can help achieve it.

How is this achieved in reality? Sometimes, it helps for survivors to describe what their **"If only…"** monster looks like once they have taken it out of their body and placed it on their shoulder. The most important part of the technique is the next part: when they come up with three or four things they would like to say to their monster to begin defeating it. Here are some typical commands:

"It's happened, and there's nothing anyone can do about it!"

"Shut up! Get out of my life. I'm moving on!"

"Go and take a running jump! And I hope you kill yourself!"

"I'll give you more than 'if only…', if you don't shut it!"

(And you can add ruder and more explicit commands…)

As with other techniques, it is helpful if the technique is practised right away. Then, continue practising it about 10–12 times per week for several weeks. This will make sure the power and control are transferred back from "the monster" to yourself.

"Finally, I got rid of my 'If only …' monster"

A man in his late twenties walked out of a good, well-paying job after an argument with his boss. He was unemployed for a while and was living in very reduced circumstances. His **"If only** …" monster spoke as follows:

- "If only you hadn't had such a late night before, you wouldn't have been so tired and irritable, when you spoke to your boss",
- "If only you had kept your mouth shut when your boss made that provocative remark!", and
- "If only I had walked away!"

By going through the procedure above, and practising it whenever the "monster" spoke, the man was able to move on. Eventually, he found another job with another company within the same industry.

8. **Write, read, and burn (or write, read, and shred)**[d]

Based on a technique from the Milwaukee Brief Therapy Centre, this exercise aims to resolve any negative memories that are intruding upon and constricting the person's present life in the form of intrusive thoughts or images.

The instructions are as follows:

A. First, write down the details of the memory, thought, or image that troubles you.

B. Now, write down any feelings you have about the memory, thought, or image. If another person is involved in the memory, address these feelings to that person, where appropriate. Include anything you would like to say or wish you could say to that person.

C. Next, re-read what you have written, reading it aloud.[e]

D. Finally, once you have done so, burn or shred the pages.

---

[d] With full acknowledgement to Yvonne Dolan and Charlie Johnson for the original version.

[e] While not essential, sometimes it is helpful psychologically to have another person present (e.g. a friend, relation, or counsellor) to hear what you read and witness the burning or shredding of the pages.

9. "Park it... and move on..."

This is a powerful instruction to the mind for dealing with intrusive thoughts; this technique is a simple statement that acknowledges the incident without attempting to bury it in any way. This has been of great help to survivors in both civilian and military contexts.

As a car-parking metaphor, it is helpful because the survivor can picture parking an old car anywhere they choose—a lay-by, car park, roadside, etc.—then walking away from it and moving on along their life journey.

They may choose to return to the car, from time to time, to take a fresh look at it, maybe sit inside for a while, or drive it around a little. In either case, they can park it again, lock it up, move on, and return to their walk along life's journey.

This metaphor is powerful in another way. What happens to cars when they are left parked up and neglected for a long time? They become dusty, covered in cobwebs, the tyres deflate, and the brakes and clutch plates rust and seize up. Eventually, they become a rusty heap, fit only for scrap—and certainly, after many years, not something you would want to revisit anyway. By this time, a great distance has been covered between the "parked" car and your life journey. What happens is that, although the car was an important part of your life, its potential to affect you in the present gradually weakens. It begins to become but a distant memory.

It is helpful for the survivor to practise saying the command, **"Park it… and move on…"**—repeating it 10 to 12 times per week when unwelcome thoughts occur, and continuing for a number of weeks afterwards to thoroughly bed-in the technique.

10. "Let it go… Let it go… Let it go…"

This technique is very powerful for dealing with intrusive thoughts. Rather than trying to push down the unpleasant thought when they arise—which, as is well known, *does not work*—the survivor is given the following instruction:

1. Acknowledge, briefly, the unpleasant thought.
2. Accept that it is unwelcome and not wanted.
3. Say to yourself, quietly but firmly:

"Let it go… Let it go… Let it go…"

This simple technique is widely used to great effect by thousands of survivors. In situations where the worker is suggesting the survivor experiment with the technique between appointments, it has proved helpful for the worker to encourage the survivor to practise it in the session, to check for appropriate emphasis and pauses.

11. "Fast-forwarding the live stream of your life"

Fast forwarding the **live stream** is used to

- bypass problem thinking,
- create a context for setting well-formed goals,
- encourage expectations of change,
- get information about *how* you can make progress, and
- find out about things you can do, which will get you to where you want to be.

Fast-forwarding the live stream of your life

Before counsellors or therapists ask this question, it is important to first gain a sufficient understanding of the survivor's current difficulties or problem situation.

Next, it is helpful to ask what type of device they usually use to watch a video (phone, laptop, iPad, etc.)

Next, it is crucial to get their full attention before asking the question. This is best achieved by adopting a slight air of mystery and then asking, "Can I ask you a rather unusual question…?" In my 30 years of asking this question as a therapist, I have yet to encounter someone say "No, you can't!" After all, as human beings, we are too curious!

Once they have agreed to the question being asked, ensure you *lower your tone of voice* and *slow down your pace of speech.* This is important.

Then, when you have their full attention, ask:

"Just imagine… you are watching a video of your life… It is the present time, and you can see all the difficulties and problems you are going through at the moment.

Then, you touch "fast-forward" and then "pause" at a point in the future when things are better… You touch "play" again…

As the video resumes… what do you notice on the screen that will let you know that your whole life situation is better?

(Remain still and quiet.)

…What else will we see…?	What else…?
…What will you be doing differently?	What else will you be doing…?
…What different reactions might you see in those closest to you…?	…What else…?
…How will your thinking have changed?	How else…?

Some people find the "fast-forwarding the video" question easier to use than others. It requires patience and some creative thinking to get a clear picture of something to do that is realistic, achievable, and measurable—something they truly want to happen.

"I kicked into touch, both the booze and the cigs"

An ex-serviceman, who had been deployed in four theatres of operations over a 7-year career, was medically discharged due to alcoholism. He had received detox treatment only before leaving the service. He was referred to an NHS community mental health team for help. The welfare worker found him living in poverty in a small filthy flat. Ashtrays piled with cigarette ends, empty wine and spirits bottles littered most surfaces, and he was in a neglected and disheveled state.

When asked the fast-forwarding the video question, he answered:

"I will have got control of all this drinking…" "I will have sorted my life out…"

"I will have this place (looking around) tidied up…"

What else…?:

"The smoking: I'll be down to no more than 5 a-day…"

"Maybe, too, I'll have spoken to those in that help office, at the Regeneration Project…"

And what else…?:

"I can't see myself working yet, but maybe I'll have a few ideas…"

"And… I'll have sorted my head out more, so I won't need the drink to block it out…Doesn't work for long anyway."

12. Ways to deal with anger build-ups

Anger is a common result of severe traumatic experiences and is quite normal and understandable. However, it can become a problem if not dealt with (i.e. get it out of the way safely, as it starts to build up). Anger outbursts can have a catastrophic effect on both property and relationships.

First, we must recognise it. Second, we need to develop a plan of action to deal with it in a safe, healthy, and controlled way.

In the following pages, you will find some ideas and techniques to help express anger safely and effectively.

There are six main ways:

I. *Chat to a (trusted) friend, colleague, counsellor, or therapist*

"A problem shared is a problem halved" is the main principle that works here. Talking to someone you can trust—who will keep what you say confidential—can provide great relief and help release any anger build-up.

II. *Write it down*

Many thousands of survivors of traumatic experiences have found it very helpful to write down emerging feelings of anger, listing how and from where they have arisen. It is important to write as much as needed, which can be done on a writing pad, in a journal, or a personal diary.

Survivors must be encouraged to take great care to keep it confidential. If it is written on loose leaf paper, there is always the option to burn or shred it afterwards. If a journal or personal diary is used, make sure it is kept in a safe and secure place. It is important to be careful what is committed to paper, just in case secrecy and confidentiality are compromised. Using a personal code or abbreviations can be helpful when referring to people, places, and events.

III. *Do some strenuous physical exercise*

Many people have found that strenuous physical exercise has a positive, discharging effect on any anger build-ups. This might involve a workout at the gym, a circuit training round, kicking a football, going for a long cycle ride, jogging, using a punchbag, or any other harmless activity. When anger builds up, it is best to keep away from others until we have found our own way to discharge it safely. (Being in the presence of others, however close they are to us, can be provocative.) Arguments may arise that can lead to anger spilling over onto people we love or hold dear, often in unhealthy or damaging ways.

When encouraging survivors to use this technique, it is helpful for them to explain to those closest to them their need to be alone at these times to get on with their chosen workout. Once those closest to you understand this, the majority become more supportive of it. Some couples, have a particular code word they use to signal the need for personal space and time and to commit to their chosen method.

"Boxercise circuits"

A soldier who carried much anger about certain situations he had been involved in while serving in the second Gulf War found it really helpful to do a couple of rounds of "boxercise" circuits in the gym whenever his anger builds up. His code word to his wife at these times was "build-up". She would reply "okay", and all would be fine once he returned.

Sec. 3

IV. *Find somewhere safe to shout it out!*

Many survivors of severe trauma and stress find it very helpful to shout out—as loudly as they can or need to—about the things that have made them feel angry about a traumatic situation(s) they experienced. So, to avoid alarming others(!)—especially those close to them—it is important to find a safe, isolated place where they can have a good shout!

Some good examples of such places are

- in a parked car, in an isolated spot, with all windows shut firmly,
- along a coastal path or on a beach,
- along a footpath in open country, in between large fields,
- in an open moorland or mountainous area, and
- in a sound-proofed room or building,

"My so-called best mate"

A travelling salesman, whose "best mate" had dated his partner while he was away working, was furious at both his partner and his so-called "best mate". He wanted the relationship to get back on track and still wanted to be friends with his mate. He knew that, initially, it would be unwise and unsafe to "have it out" with each of them. So, to safely discharge the overwhelming anger, he parked his car in a lay-by on a rarely used country road and shouted at them in their absence. He told another mate: "I was quite hoarse when I'd finished, but I felt better!"

A few sessions later, he was able to speak calmly to both of them individually without risking violence.

V. *Draw it or paint it*

Some survivors have more artistic leanings and find either drawing or painting very therapeutic. Many find these as good ways to discharge anger (and other negative) feelings.

VI. *Play your choice of music loudly*

Playing music loudly can be an effective way to connect with and release strong, angry feelings. It might be a particular track or a whole album. This can be done at home, in the car, or through a personal sound system (NB: Be mindful not to disturb neighbours or damage your eardrums!).

How to measure the discharge of negative feelings

One effective way to measure how well you are doing is to use the "solution-focused feelings tank", as shown in Figure 1.

First, it is important to explain how the tank can be used. It is shaped like a garden water butt, containing the amount of a strong negative feeling you may be feeling at

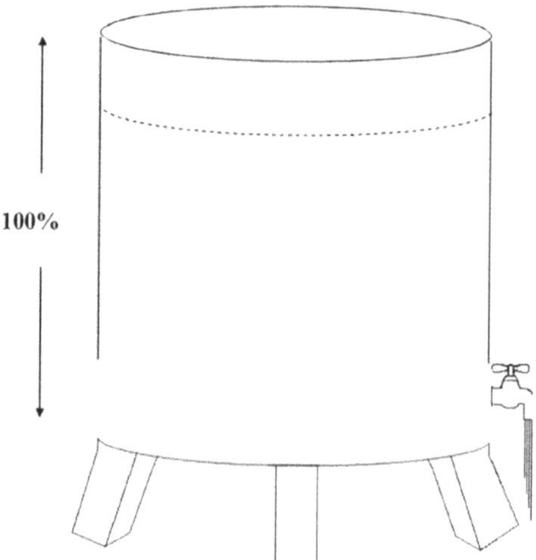

Figure 1. The solution-focused feelings tank.

the moment (e.g. anger, frustration, disappointment, sadness, shame, guilt, and regret).

The explanation about how to use it is as follows:

1. "There is no inlet pipe, but there is a tap over that you can control."
2. "You may never completely empty the feelings tank about this situation (i.e. anger in this case) because the tap is positioned higher than the bottom of the tank."
3. "How much emotion—let's say anger—have you managed to release through this tap so far?" (Suppose it is 3%.)

4. "That's 3%! How have you managed to do that!?"
5. "What's the next small step you could take to run off another 1% over the next 2–3 weeks?"
6. "And what else could you do to reduce the level by another 1%?"

   … and so on.

This exercise has proven very helpful in empowering survivors to take control of the negative feelings that keep surfacing as unwanted thoughts. It is also a very affirming exercise, as only occasionally does someone answer that their tank is 100 percent full. Majority of people initially respond with levels between 70 percent and 95 percent. So, some credit can be given for what actions/changes in thinking they have already made.

13. Change your mental attitude towards unwelcome thoughts

- It is the way we respond to unwelcome thoughts that causes us distress.
- It is our reaction that enables these thoughts to have power and influence over us.
- The more we try to push unwelcome thoughts away, the more they will struggle to get back into our conscious mind (e.g. Notice what happens when

you tell yourself: "Whatever you do, *do not* think of pink elephants!")

- To prevent ourselves from being pestered by unwelcome thoughts, we need to use an effective technique to reduce their frequency.

Survivors can be helped by the following four-step approach to changing your mental attitude:

1. Welcome the intrusive thought (or fear).
2. Imagine a cartoon character (e.g. Tom Cat from Tom and Jerry, or Donald Duck).
3. Give it a squeaky voice.
4. Have the cartoon character speak out the thought (e.g. "Remember that car crash where you slowed down but didn't stop to help the injured?").

The result of the cartoon imagery is to reprogramme the initial fearful emotional reaction, effectively taking out the power it once held over you. The less you fear the thought, the less likely it is to occur during the day. In turn, the emotional reaction will be neutralised.

14. Visualisation

This is done best when either sitting or standing and should last for 10 to 15 minutes. When practised daily for a few weeks, it achieves the objective of enabling the survivor to regain control over anxious or unwanted thoughts. When performed immediately after technique 10, it has even more power over anxious thoughts or any kind.

The mind needs to regularly release what it is holding on to. When it does, soothing and beneficial results can be achieved.

With practice, this technique enables you to release all stress within minutes of starting the exercise. You will have trained your brain. Daily practice before bedtime also enables you to sleep more soundly.

Survivors can follow the following instructions:

i. In either a sitting or standing position, gently shift your attention to your breath.
ii. Place one hand on your stomach and the other on your upper chest.
iii. Take in a breath, allowing your stomach to expand forward as you do so, and let it fall back on the out-breath. (Your hand on your chest should have no or little movement.)
iv. Repeat this three times, lengthening the in-breath to the count of 7 and the out-breath to the count of 11. (This is called 7/11 diaphragmatic breathing and is referred to in other parts of this book.) The more you practise 7/11 breathing, the stronger

your diaphragm will become, and the more naturally it will function.[f]

v. Now, slow your breathing down even more by adding a short pause after the out-breath, before breathing in again. (At first, you might feel you are not getting enough air but with practice, you will become more comfortable with it).

vi. If any unwanted or unwelcome thoughts arise as you do this, simply let them go on the out-breath and focus back to your breathing.

vii. Next, shift your attention to your feet and try to really feel them. See if you can feel each toe, one-by-one.

viii. Now, visualise the soles of your feet with roots growing slowly downwards, deep into the earth beneath. Visualise the roots growing more quickly and firmly, so that you are now rooted to the spot like a magnificent oak tree.

ix. Concentrate on this feeling of being grounded securely and safely for a minute or so.

x. Now, visualise a cloud of bright light forming up high above you.

---

[f] Wisegeek. What is the Diaphragm Muscle? www.wisegeek.com/what-is-the-diaphragm- muscle.htm (accessed 22 May 2017).

xi. Notice now a bolt of lightning shooting down from the cloud onto the top of your head. As it does, it transforms itself into a circular band of white light, which slowly descends from your head, past your shoulders, waist, and legs, all the way down to your toes. As it moves downward, feel it clearing away any rubbish you may have been thinking about, leaving you with a clear and free mental state.

xii. Repeat this image of the circular band of light passing down your body for about five times, until you feel a sense of all anxious thoughts being cleared away and released.

xiii. Now, visualise yourself standing under a large, luminescent waterfall where you are able to breathe easily.

- o The water is bubbling, radiant, cleansing, and full of vitality.
- o Feel the water washing down your body, soothing and calming you as it does.
- o Hear the splash of the water on the ground around you.
- o As you enjoy this experience even more, tell yourself that not only is the water life itself, but

Sec. 3

it is also washing away any anxiety, stress, or worry from both your mind and your body.

xiv.   After a few moments, and in your own time, open your eyes. Then, gently and slowly move away to what you were doing before or want to do next. (As you move away, avoid ripping too much of the ground away, as each root is severed!)

This visualisation, like many others, achieves the twin objective of restoring calm and replacing a sense of lack of control, with one of *control*.

15. The solution-focused feelings tank (See Figure 1)

Sometimes, an intrusive thought is connected to a negative feeling we have about a situation. This negative feeling can be any one or several of the following:

Anger	Hurt	Self-blame
Disappointment	Being overwhelmed	Grief
		Worthlessness
Fear	Rage	Confusion
Guilt	Regret	Embarrassment
Sadness	Worry	Low self-
Shame	Helplessness	confidence, etc.

If we let them, these negative feelings can take control of us. Therefore, it is important to take back the control. Using the solution-focused feelings tank (Figure 1) is very helpful to achieve this.

Dealing with "The Lows"

1. Work at and maintain a good, balanced diet
2. Drink plenty of liquids
3. Remind yourself of the power of humour
4. Do something pleasurable for the simple joy of doing it
5. Build up your physical fitness or a sufficient level of physical activity
6. Keep self-confidence and self-esteem at a high level
7. See "the lows" as a virus that can be dealt with
8. Get out there and reconnect with supportive people
9. Acknowledge to yourself that you're experiencing a touch of "the lows"

10. Increase your knowledge/get more information
11. Get enough sleep
12. The "rainy-day letter"
13. "Don't just lie there, get up!"
14. Breathe your way to a relaxed state
15. What to do if you let "the lows" get too low

One thing is for certain: all survivors will have low days as they make their journey back to full recovery and control. The good news is that, as the tools and techniques in this book are mastered, you will be more in control, more often. This means you will not be controlled by negative thinking and the "lows" accompanying them. However, it is not realistic to think you can prevent all low days. There will be times when you feel you are not getting anywhere, asking questions such as, "What is it all about anyway?", "I feel just like giving up!", or "I feel I'm back at square one!". It is most helpful to have a plan or strategy ready for days like these. Some practical techniques are as follows:

1. Work at and maintain a good, balanced diet

As we are resolving reactions to past events, there can be a tendency to "comfort eat".

This does us no favours at all. Nor does it do any favours to our family and friends, who have to cope with our reduced agility, poorer health, and lower energy levels.

The trouble is that comfort eating tends to consist mainly of all the wrong things: chocolates, sweets, biscuits, fast food, and fizzy drinks.

Contrary to some opinions, healthy eating need not be expensive. In fact, it can often be cheaper. Ensure you get your "5-a-day" fruits and vegetables. A healthy intake of the whole range of vitamins and minerals helps towards our overall well-being. It is sensible to cut down on saturated fats, salt, and sugar too.

2. Drink plenty of liquids

Ensuring 2–3 litres of fluids in various forms every day will help you feel better and support your brain and body to function as they should. Headaches, too, can be avoided. A car engine running on little oil will not perform as well as when the dipstick shows "full". Drinking water is preferable, but fruit juice, squash, or hot beverages are okay too. With the last three, however, care should be taken to avoid taking in too much sugar or caffeine—neither of which is healthy.

3. Remind yourself of the power of humour

Usually, a good sign that we are feeling low is that our sense of humour fades. Answer: get it going again! Do this by watching a comic DVD, Internet searching for humorous websites, watching cat videos on YouTube, or reading a joke book.

Laughter is a good antidote to feeling low. There is plenty of evidence showing that the chemicals released into the bloodstream by laughter help us feel better.

4. Do something pleasurable for the simple joy of doing it

Everyone has their preferred way(s) of deriving personal pleasure or satisfaction. If space allowed, I could list over 1,000 here! Although you might not feel up to doing it right now, you will feel the benefit of doing something pleasurable anyway.

5. Build up your physical fitness or a sufficient level of physical activity

Fit body—fit mind. Everyone can do something to improve their level of physical fitness or physical activity. It is a good daily discipline to develop.

It can range from a full marathon or a "boxercise" workout in the gym to gentle arm swinging and arm and waist tensioning from a chair—and all points in between.

Again, a lot of scientific evidence is out there to prove how we can feel better when we get involved in some form of exercise, whether "high-burn" or gentle.

6. Keep self-confidence and self-esteem at a high level

Self-confidence and self-esteem are interconnected. If we have feelings about having little personal value, our confidence is low, too. Similarly, if we feel low in confidence, we won't be able to value ourselves as much.

The answer is to tackle either one or the other, in order to boost both.

"I live in this village"

A road crash victim had been both withdrawn and isolated from others in his village for many months. He lacked the confidence to go out, having a whole collection of helpers who would bring things to him. Walking was painful due to the extent of injuries he sustained in the crash. Also, he had a slight limp. In addition to his low self-confidence, his self-esteem was low too; he felt worthless, believing he had nothing to contribute to anyone.

With the help of a supportive friend, he was able to tell himself:

"I have every right to walk around the village. I survived that crash in which others died and can hold my head up high. Going for a short walk in the evening will help build my confidence for a longer walk tomorrow."

Result: eventually, he was able to walk in the village on most days and got to know other villagers better. He was invited to play in a local skittles team, built up his social life, spent 2 days a week in voluntary work, and was thinking of meeting up with a local careers advisor regarding future paid employment opportunities.

7. See "the lows" as a virus that can be dealt with

"The lows" virus finds a good breeding ground if both our confidence and self-esteem are low; we are feeling "stressed-out", physically run down, suppressing our thoughts and feelings, or full of anger and resentment. *Anyone* can find themselves in this situation at some point in their life. These feelings are normal and are not a sign of 'depression'. [The serotonin deficit theory of depression has now been debunked (Moncrieff, J. 2022).]

The important thing to do to defend against or defeat this virus is to work hard at all the techniques in this section. Once achieved, the results will be

- clearer thinking,
- improved sense of humour,
- higher self-confidence and self-esteem,
- better mood, and
- higher energy levels.

8. Get out there and reconnect with supportive people

Withdrawal and isolation are common results of "the lows". Even though it may seem very hard or nearly impossible, it is vital to reconnect—with old workmates, friends from the past, relatives, friendly neighbours—in fact, anyone supportive whom you can talk to and confide in with ease.

The principle that operates is: "A problem shared is a problem halved!" Tell yourself it is okay to talk about your thoughts and feelings with people you trust, even if you were told some time ago that this was not permitted. Once you have done this, notice the difference it makes to how you feel about yourself.

9. Acknowledge to yourself that you're experiencing a touch of "the lows"

...then, take action

Often, *anything* constructive we do can get us back to feeling okay again. The domino effect applies. It does not matter what we do—giving ourselves a good talking-to, taking up some physical activity, writing down our thoughts, ideas, and feelings about the situation, listening to inspiring music, or talking to someone we trust—can trigger a ripple effect.

10. Increase your knowledge/get more information

Searching the Internet, reading booklets or pamphlets, and discussing with a friend or colleague can all help increase our knowledge about "the lows" and how to tackle them. People used to feel they were going mad or "losing it" before they realised that it is a normal and understandable situation to get in when we do not take a mentally healthy approach to things.

11. Get enough sleep

It is not the quantity of sleep that is important, but *quality*. When unresolved thoughts go around and around in our minds, it is hard to get into deep sleep. It may be difficult to get off to sleep, return to sleep after waking during the night, or you may wake up very early. Sometimes, even after sleeping for nine hours, if it has not been of sufficient quality, we may awaken tired and feeling exhausted.

(For many, many tips and ideas for improving sleep, see Section 5).

12. The "rainy-day letter[a]"

While some of life's difficult passages are impossible to anticipate, thankfully, they are not impossible to prepare for. That is the purpose of "the rainy-day letter". It can function as a bridge over life's chasms, not in the sense of providing numbing or "faking" the experience, but rather as a way to help transform difficult moments into experiences of mastery and hope. It is ironic that the very times when one most needs to remember their strengths and resources are often those occasions when it is easiest to forget them. The "rainy-day letter" or, if you prefer, "rainy-day postcard" is a way to remind us of these strengths and resources at exactly those times when they are most needed.

[a] Yvonne Dolan, M.A. Charlie Johnson, M.S.W. Copyright 1995 Excerpted from Dolan, Y., 1998. *Beyond Survival: Living Well is the Best Revenge*. Reproduced with permission.

The instructions are as follows:

How to make your own "rainy-day letter"

This is a letter from you to you. It should be written not in a moment of despair, but in a moment of relative calm and well-being. It is an emotional insurance policy against the inevitability of those darker moments that come at various times in life—a sort of "emergency roadside repair kit" for the spirit. The letter should contain, but is not limited to, the following:

- a list of nurturing activities to do,
- a list of nurturing people to call,
- reminders of your positive character traits,
- reminders of spiritual or philosophical beliefs that strengthen you,
- reminders of some of your dreams and hopes for the future,
- special advice or other reminders important to you.

Once completed, put your rainy-day letter somewhere you can easily find it when needed. Some people like to make several copies—one to carry in a wallet, briefcase, or purse; another to keep in a special drawer or car's glove compartment, and so on.

13. "Don't just lie there, get up!"

When we wake up in the morning and just continue lying there, the mind goes into overdrive—it starts working on the issues and concerns in our life. These issues and concerns can then seem ten times worse than when we are up and walking around.

When keeping it simple, a chemical process starts in the brain and the body, releasing bad chemicals into our system. These start flowing through our arteries, with unpleasant results.

It is important, in cases where survivors have fallen into this habit, to experiment and observe the differences and benefits of getting up and getting going, rather than just lying there.

14. Breathe your way to a relaxed state

Find somewhere comfortable to sit or lie. Then, with your eyes lightly closed, empty your mind of all current thoughts. Now, take a short, slow breath in, and then breathe out slowly and steadily for the count of 11. Hold it for about 2 seconds. Then, breathe in again for the count of 7. Repeat this for about six or seven times. The more controlled and deliberate you are, the deeper your sense of relaxation will be. To maintain the good effects for some time afterwards, wait a few minutes before slowly and carefully getting up and moving on to another activity. (This is the 7/11 diaphragmatic breathing described in earlier sections.)

15. What to do if you let "the lows" get too low

Sometimes, while going through a period of "the lows", we can let a situation spiral downwards. This is unpleasant, to say the least, as those of us who have been there can testify. Should this happen, call a "Halt!" immediately, promising yourself that you will take the first small step back—*and* within the next hour.

Should you be feeling so low that suicidal thoughts and ideas enter your mind? Know that there are many options available and that you can take. One of these is to read through the many tools and techniques in my book (see Henden, 2017) on preventing suicidal thoughts. Another is to speak to a professional you know and can trust. Close friends or organisations such as The Samaritans can also provide support.

Remember: suicide is never the solution to what may seem an unsolvable problem. Know that help is available and you are not alone.

Section

Dealing with Sleep Disturbance

PART ONE

A. Techniques for Preparing for Bed

1. Read a book
2. Have some cereal or a milky drink
3. Watch a happy or boring film
4. Establish a routine
5. Get enough exercise
6. Eat early
7. Prepare well for bedtime
8. Open the window a little
9. Use lavender oil
10. Listen to a story
11. Complete some tasks

12. Turn off the late news
13. Sort out your curtains
14. Resolve disagreements
15. Go for mattress comfort
16. Alternate quilts for the seasons
17. Go for softer/harder pillows
18. Drink relaxing teas
19. Put your worries on hold
20. Buy some earplugs
21. Steer clear of caffeine and chocolate
22. Undress slowly for bed
23. "Larks" and "owls" help each other
24. Reduce emotional and psychological stress

B. Getting Off to Sleep

1. Lie flat and stare
2. Count sheep
3. Use reverse psychology
4. Turn your pillow
5. Tense and then relax your muscles
6. Count backwards
7. Read through the whole of this subsection
8. Listen through headphones
9. Go for absolute stillness

10. **Relax your shoulders**
11. **Worry not**
12. **Visualise calm scenes**
13. **Practise 7/11 breathing**
14. **Relax your jaws**

C. Getting Back to Sleep, if Waking or Awakened in the Night

1. **Think relaxing words**
2. **Make a list of worrying thoughts**
3. **Use your favourite guided fantasy**
4. **Tell yourself sleep does not matter**
5. **Watch some TV**
6. **Get up and read**
7. **Pray for people**
8. **Forgive right now**
9. **Turn your quilt**
10. **Get up and do it right now**
11. **Crawl into a "safe and secure" tunnel**
12. **Use the 5-4-3-2-1 method**
13. **Five girls' names**

It is important for us to talk through, or in some way, resolve traumatic or disturbing memories and thoughts during our waking hours. If we do not do this, or if we try to suppress them with drugs or alcohol, our brain will get stuck in these memories and thoughts overnight, while we are asleep. This can be the stuff of nightmares. We can be awakened by this activity and may find it difficult to get back to sleep. The main purpose of dreaming is to try and resolve the unresolved conflicts of the day. It is better, then, to try and resolve as many conflicts as we can during our waking hours. That is what Sections 1—4 have been about.

Prevention is better than cure. It is better if we sort out conflicts and painful memories by using the tools and techniques outlined in the previous sections. Moreover, in the following pages are some tips and techniques for:

- preparing for bed,
- getting off to sleep, and
- getting back to sleep if awakened by disturbing dreams.

The following tips are addressed directly to survivors from anywhere on the spectrum of severe trauma and stress. Anyone can try them out for effectiveness—whether trauma survivors or not. When practitioners try these tips for themselves, they are more likely to recommend them to others.

A. Techniques for Preparing for Bed

It is helpful to create a "no-man's land" between day and night. This can be done by preparing for bedtime at least half an hour before getting into bed.

1. Read a book

A good way to empty our minds of all the cares and concerns of the day is to read an easygoing book, last thing at night.

2. Have some cereal or a milky drink

Many have found that a bowl of cereal or a milky drink before going to bed is helpful. This helps with digestion and diverts blood from the thinking brain.

3. Watch a happy or boring film

Watching a happy or even a boring film before going to bed puts a line under the day's cares and helps you prepare for sleep. Some television programmes can have the same effect.

4. Establish a soothing routine

Within half to one hour before going to bed, do a soothing routine that suits you best. This might involve having a soak in a hot bath, listening to your favourite music, working at a jig-saw puzzle, and so on.

5. Get enough exercise

Make sure each day is well balanced with adequate mental and physical exercise. Energetic exercise at some points during the day has many benefits. Gentle exercise, taken an hour or so after an evening meal, also promotes relaxation and aids digestion. There are some mobile phone apps to help and encourage you with this.

6. Eat early

Eat your evening meal at least one and a half to two hours before bedtime. This helps avoid the "heaviness" that can be felt after a large meal while trying to go off to sleep. Drinking too much alcohol with a meal can slow digestion and increase that feeling of heaviness.

7. Prepare well for bedtime

Avoid exciting, dynamic, or focused activities during the late evening. Also, avoid intense discussions or phone calls at least two hours before bedtime.

8. Open the window a little

Opening your bedroom window slightly to maintain a fresh air supply throughout the night can prevent "stuffiness", thereby reducing the risk of night-time waking. Also, it prevents carbon dioxide concentrations, which can rise as much as 70 percent by morning. A room temperature that is not too hot and not too cold will aid deeper sleep, too.

9. Use lavender oil

Drops of lavender oil on your pillow can help you relax before drifting off to sleep.

10. Listen to a story

Getting immersed in a bedtime radio story or play is a good way of preparing for sleep.

11. Complete some tasks

Think of some tasks during the day that, if you started or completed them, would help you sleep that night (e.g. tax form, application form, loose shelving bracket, loose carpet, etc.).

12. Turn off the late news

As television and radio news, selected for listeners, tends mainly to focus on bad news, this can affect both sleep and dream work. You are better off listening to it earlier in the day. Listening to, as opposed to watching the news, is less likely to disturb sleep, too. One survivor said, "I listen to the 6 pm news, but not the 10 p.m."

13. Sort out your curtains

Buy some heavier curtains or have your existing ones lined. Make sure all gaps are covered to prevent chinks of early morning light shining through. This is especially important during the summer months.

14. Resolve disagreements

It is helpful, where possible, to sort out any daytime disagreements you might have with family members or friends before going to bed. Resolved disagreements are good for settled sleep.

15. Go for mattress comfort

It is helpful to ensure your bed is the most comfortable for you. Some people prefer softer mattresses to others. A good mattress is not necessarily the most expensive. It is important to pay attention to this, as we spend approximately one-quarter to one-third of our lives in bed. If the mattress is unsatisfactory in some way, a quick-fix or cheaper option is to lay an old quilt or piece of foam under the bottom sheet.

16. Alternate quilts with the seasons

If using a quilt, it is important to make sure the tog rating is right for you and the season. If finances permit, alternate between summer and winter quilts to maintain good night-time body temperature.

17. Go for softer/harder pillows

Changing your pillows to softer, harder, or more comfortable ones can be pleasant for both your face and head. Try experimenting with two thin pillows or one thicker one.

18. Drink relaxing teas

Have a cup of herbal tea, such as chamomile, lemon verbena, lemon balm, or peppermint, before going to bed. Alternatively, sipping warm water can have a similar effect.

19. Put your worries on hold

Before going to bed, write down your worries, troubles, or mental conflicts in a notebook or a notepad for action tomorrow or at a definite future date. It can be more effective to put a heading on the page with the exact date and time when you will give them some thought.

20. Buy some earplugs

Fitting a suitable pair of earplugs can block out all but the loudest noises that might wake you during your sleep. They are especially useful for light sleepers. Finding the right type to suit you is important, as some are more comfortable than others. This is important if you live near a busy road, railway, or under an airport flight path. Two of the most popular types are condensed-shaped foam and the wax barrel-shaped ones. Many prefer to cut the latter type in half before moulding them to fit. Surprisingly (and thankfully!), while even the most effective earplugs screen out most noise, they do not seem to be effective against smoke alarms, fire alarms and alarm clocks!

21. Steer clear of caffeine and chocolate

The stimulants in strong tea, coffee, and chocolate are likely to delay your getting off to sleep. Keeping them out of your diet at least five hours prior to bedtime can be helpful. Some people find that chilies, black pepper, mustard, and strong spices eaten with food after 5 p.m. can cause midnight waking.

22. Undress slowly for bed

Taking your time—plenty of time—to remove each item of clothing before sliding into bed can help your body cool down better for sleeping.

23. "Larks" and "owls" help each other

If you are a "lark", and your spouse is an "owl", it is most likely you will be first to bed on nearly all occasions. As a "lark", a request for your "owl" to enter the bedroom and get into bed quietly when they come in late will reduce the risk of waking you. On the other hand, if you are an "owl", ask your "lark" to get out of bed slowly and quietly when they wake early in the morning, so as not to disturb your sleep.

24. Reduce emotional and psychological stress

Avoid putting yourself under too much pressure. Doing so helps keep your stress levels within acceptable limits and, as a result, you are more likely to sleep better. You may need to say "no" more often.

B. Getting Off to Sleep

1. Lie flat and stare

Lie flat on your back and stare at a spot on the ceiling. Try to keep your eyelids open and still, avoiding blinking, for as long as possible. Although it does not matter if you do blink from time to time, continue staring at your chosen point on the ceiling.

2. Count sheep

This is probably the most well-known. It works best when you concentrate hard on the activity, taking it very seriously. Count your sheep—both on a hillside and out across the meadow, and wherever else you can see them: "Two by the gate, one by the round bush, three by the stream", and so on.

3. Use "reverse" psychology

Try to stay awake for as long as you can. Be as sincere and determined as possible with this. It helps if you tell yourself it does not matter if you do not sleep—you are resting anyway by lying flat. Many find they fall asleep sooner rather than later using this method.

4. Turn your pillow

If your head feels too warm from overthinking, try turning your pillow over to the "cold side".

5. Tense and then relax your muscles

Beginning with your jaws, gently tense the muscles and relax them before moving through the rest of your body, right down to your feet. As a result, you will feel a slight heaviness, calmness, and a sense of relaxation. This promotes deeper sleep.

6. Count backwards

Very slowly, count backwards in your head by threes, from 301 down to 1.

7. Read through the whole of this subsection

If you are having difficulty sleeping, there is no better read! Choose the part you want to make use of tonight.

8. Listen through headphones

Listening softly to the radio or music through headphones creates a barrier between you and everything "outside". As you begin to feel sleepy, simply slide off the headphones and press the "off" switch on your radio or music system.

9. Go for absolute stillness

Lie on your back, very, very still, without moving a muscle. Gently resist any temptation to move. Empty your mind of all concerns and think pleasant thoughts only. Through the stillness, sleepiness can take over.

10. Relax your shoulders

Consciously lowering your shoulders away from your earlobes can help release the tensions of the day. First, lower your shoulders and let them return to a comfortable position. Then lower them again. Let them return once more, and lower them again.

11. Worry not

When worries about the future come to mind, tell yourself that you will deal with them in the coming days and weeks. Often, our worries revolve around things that may *never* happen.

12. Visualise calm scenes

When we visualise some of our favourite calm scenes, examining each carefully in detail, it distracts us from life's cares and helps us relax.

13. Practise 7/11 breathing

This is a powerful technique for regaining control of both our body and mind, which has been featured in earlier sections. Simply breathe out through your mouth for the count of 11, ensuring your abdomen contracts as you do so. Then, when all the breath is exhaled, allow your diaphragm to pull down as you breathe in slowly through your nose for the count of 7. When done correctly, *the abdomen extends, and the chest remains still.* This is important and may require practice to get it right. The result will be calmness and a greater sense of control over both body and mind.

14. Relax your jaws

Focusing on your jaw muscles, relaxing them, and allowing your mouth to hang open is an effective way to reduce tension.

C. Getting Back to Sleep, if Waking or Awakened in the Night

1. Think relaxing words

Say to yourself slowly and quietly, in your own mind, the following words:

"Calmness. . ."   "Sleepiness..."   "Drowsiness..."
"Relaxation..."   "Heaviness..."   "Tranquillity..."
"Serenity..."   "Peace..."   "Sweet Dreams..."

You can add other relaxing words. Then, say them even more slowly and repeat many times for as long as necessary.

2. Make a list of worrying thoughts

Sometimes, worries, regrets, sadness, and unresolved conflicts from the day can awaken us in the form of vivid dreams or nightmares. This is a natural process, though it can be unpleasant when it happens. Without turning on the light, it helps to list them on a piece of paper or notepad at your bedside as soon as you realise what has woken you. It is important to promise that you will act on them tomorrow, making some progress towards resolving them or coming to terms with them in some way. The process of writing them down like this seems to satisfy the brain, recognising that you have a plan for dealing with them. This technique can be even more effective if the notepad or piece of paper is headed with something like: "THINGS TO THINK ABOUT AT 8:00 AM".

3. Use your favourite guided fantasy

Transport yourself to your favourite place (a hillside, meadow, beach, far-off island, etc.). Call to mind five things you can see, five things you can hear, five things you can smell, five things you can taste, and five things you can touch. Concentrate hard on your favourite place, experiencing sensations such as calmness, pleasure, delight, wonder, and relaxation. Stay at your favourite place for as long as you like before drifting off to sleep. (Over 90 percent of people who use this method say they can never remember getting beyond halfway before sleep takes over!)

4. Tell yourself sleep does not matter

By saying to yourself, "I don't mind if I sleep, lie awake, or doze gently. I am getting valuable rest, either way". This can take the pressure off and thereby help you to get back to sleep. It is a form of reverse psychology.

5. Watch some boring TV

Get up to watch some trivia or something boring on night-time TV, preferably wearing minimal clothing. Return to bed when you either feel bored or too cold. The contrasting cosiness of the bed you return to will be comforting and will promote sleep.

Sec. 5

6. Get up and read

On waking in the night, get up and skim through a chapter or a few pages from an "easy-to-read" book before returning to bed. If you are alone in the bedroom, you might simply sit up in bed to read.

7. Pray for people

Praying systematically for each member of your family and your friends is purposeful, and it can also help distract you as you concentrate on the needs and worries of others.

8. Forgive right now

If you are holding a grudge or any ill-feeling towards someone, forgive them totally and unconditionally right now. This is important because the only person being damaged by such feelings, if you allow them to persist, is you. (N.B.: Forgiving someone does not necessarily mean that you have to have any type of relationship with them.)

9. Turn your quilt

By slowly and carefully turning your quilt over to the cold side, you may cool your body down sufficiently to encourage sleep. (This is best when sleeping alone, as it could become somewhat alarming to your spouse!)

Another way is to peel back the covers temporarily, allow yourself to cool down for a short while, then slowly pull the covers back over you.

10. Get up and do it now

If something you need to do (draft an email or letter, make a "to do" list, etc.) is going round and round in your head, and it's practicable, get up and do it now. Then return to bed, comforting yourself with the knowledge that it's now done and out of the way—or at least you have made a start.

11. Crawl into "a safe and secure tunnel"

Imagine you have hollowed out a small, dry tunnel in a hillside. You have furnished it with a narrow mattress, a sleeping bag, and a pillow. You have a small nightlight safely burning in the corner. You have carved small shelves into the soft rock for your little personal objects. Now, feel the sense of security and notice all you can see in your safe, cosy environment before gently drifting back to sleep.

12. Use the 5-4-3-2-1 method

Open your eyes.
Notice five things you can see.

Close your eyes.
Notice five things you can hear.
Notice five things you feel in your body (warmth, pillows, etc.; not emotions).

Open your eyes.
Notice four things you can see.

Close your eyes.
Notice four things you can hear.
Notice four things you feel in your body.

Open your eyes.
Notice three things you can see.

Close your eyes.
Notice three things you can hear.
Notice three things you feel in your body.

Open your eyes.
Notice two things you can see.

Close your eyes.
Notice two things you can hear.
Notice two things you feel in your body.

Open your eyes.
Notice one thing you can see.

Close your eyes.
Notice one thing you can hear.
Notice one thing you feel in your body.

Repeat if necessary. (It often takes two repetitions to induce sleep.)

After using the exercise four or five times, it will become easier, and its calming effect will be greater.

13. Five girls' names

Think of five girls' names beginning with A. (e.g. Andrea, Audrey, Ann, Anilese, and Agatha)

Think of five girls' names beginning with B. (e.g. Beryl, Bettina, Barbara, Beverley, and Becky)

Think of five girls' names beginning with C. (e.g. Carol, Clare, Christine, Celia, and Cordelia)

Think of five girls' names beginning with D…

And so on…

(Most people do not get beyond H before drifting off to sleep.)

Section

Living Life to the Full (or, as Full as Possible)

1. Remind yourself about your qualities, strengths, skills, resources, and other personal characteristics
2. How have you used these qualities, strengths, skills, and other attributes so far?
3. How will these qualities, strengths, and skills, and other attributes be helpful to you in the future?
4. Fast-forwarding the video of your life
5. Scaling progress on the video of your life
6. What have you done or thought about that has been helpful to you so far?
7. What have you found helpful in what others have said or done?

8. The power of small steps
9. Who are your main encouragers and/or supporters?
10. Write down your dream(s) for the future
11. Those who have "done it", whom you most admire
12. What gives your life meaning and purpose?
13. Keeping all drugs at bay
14. Seek out intimacy in relationships
15. Reconnect with yourself
16. Reconnect to a community
17. Connect to God or "a higher power"
18. Write a letter to someone you really admire
19. Kick the "PTSD" label into touch
20. The amazing effect of the first small step
21. Do not fall for the "depression" label
22. What helped you survive at the time of the incident?
23. What else helped?
24. What strengths and skills did you bring into play at the time?
25. What else have you been through in life that was difficult, and what helped you then?
26. Which of the things that helped you then could be useful to you again now?

27. Thinking of others who have gone through the same or a similar ordeal, what helped that person/those people deal with it?

28. What does it mean to you to have survived these traumatic events?

29. When these traumatic events are even less of a problem in your life, what will you be thinking about and doing instead?

30. How have the experiences and events you have gone through made you a stronger person?"

31. How have the experiences and events you have gone through made you a more determined person?

32. How do you maintain your hope that you can regain a better life in the future?

33. How will others close to you know how well you have succeeded in living life to the full?

34. What helps you most in keeping any intrusive thoughts and memories under control?

35. Which experiences of safety or comfort from the past do you make use of now?

36. What symbol of safety or comfort from the past do /could you make use of now?

37. What rituals could you perform when you have reached your goal of living life to the full? How would you celebrate?

38. How do you remain hopeful and optimistic about the future?

39. If you need more hope, how would you make that happen?

Survivors of severe trauma and stress deserve more than to know they have survived whatever incidents they have experienced or were involved in (see Appendix D: Victim–Survivor–Thriver). Survival alone is not living, but a form of existence at a lower level. "The lows" occur most often during the victim stage, and less often in the survivor stage. Thrivers experience "the lows" *far less* frequently.

Living life to the full—being as fulfilled as possible, with a maximum sense of meaning and purpose—must be our aim. Without meaning, purpose, and direction, we are simply "as straws in the wind". "Going with the flow" (or something similar) is not an option. Remember, only *dead* fish go with the flow.

Within this section, you will find some tips and techniques to help you live life to the full and thrive. Yvonne Dolan (1991, 1998) outlined the three stages of survival. It is the third stage (the authentic life/living life to the full/thriver) that we need to aspire to.

It may be that we have lost a limb (or limbs), have some degree of reduced physical functioning, or have some reduced brain capacity due to traumatic brain injury. Our hearing or sight may have been affected. While fully acknowledging these limitations, it is of great importance to strive to live life as fully as possible. We owe it to ourselves and to those closest to us. History is peppered with stories of people who have found that their limitations were not as limiting as they first thought. There are many modern-day inspiring examples too.

We know from experience that many who have been in life-threatening situations or places of extreme danger are thankful they survived upon their return. What follows are some tips, tools, and techniques for opening up the discussion about living life to the full. This section has been written as such so that it can be used as a pull-out workbook. Most survivors approach this section with enthusiasm and commitment.

Tools and Techniques

1. Remind yourself about your strengths, qualities, skills, resources, and other personal characteristics

Complete the following list:

(1)   (8)

(2)   (9)

(3)   (10)

(4)   (11)

(5)   (12)

(6)   (13)

(7)   (14)

In addition, if your best friend sat opposite you, what would they add to the above?

(1)

(2)

(3)

(4)

(5)

2. How have you used these qualities, strengths, skills, and other attributes so far?

Write down some examples of how, or in what ways, you have put some of these into practice to get to where you are today.

(a)

(b)

(c)

3. How will these qualities, strengths, skills, and other attributes be helpful to you in the future?

(Often, a good between-session task is to do the following exercise over the next 2–3 weeks.)

Using your answers to question 1, write down how some of these will be helpful to you as you face challenges, decisions, and other situations in the future.

(a)

(b)

(c)

(d)

4. "Fast-forwarding the video of your life"
(This technique also appears in Section. 3.)
Fast-forwarding the **video** is used to:

- bypass problem thinking,
- create a context for setting well-formed goals,
- encourage expectations of change,
- get information about how you can make progress, and
- find out about things you can do, which will get you to where you want to be.

Fast-forwarding the video
Before asking yourself this question, it is important to bring to mind or write down the details about your current difficulties or problem situation.

Next, ask yourself the following question:

"Just imagine… I am watching a video of my life…
Then I touch "fast-forward" and then touch "pause"
at a point in the future when things are better… I
then touch "play"…

As the video resumes, what do I notice on the screen… that will let me know that my whole life situation is better?

… What else will I see? … What else?

… What will I be doing differently? … What else will I be doing?

… What different reactions might I see in those closest to me?

… What else?

… How will my thinking have changed? … How else?

Answer:

Some people find the "fast-forwarding the video" question easier to use than others. It involves some creative thinking to get a clear picture of something to do that is realistic, achievable, measurable, and something you truly want. Work hard at this.

"I kicked into touch both the booze and the cigs"
(The same example as in Section 3)

An ex-serviceman, who had been deployed in four theatres of operations over a 7-year career was medically discharged due to "alcoholism". He had received detox treatment only before leaving the service. He was referred to an NHS community mental health team for help. The welfare worker found him living in poverty, in a small filthy flat. Ashtrays were piled high with cigarette-ends, empty wine and spirits bottles littered most surfaces, and he was in a neglected and disheveled state.

When asked the fast-forwarding the video question, he answered:

"I will have got control of all this drinking…"
"I will have sorted my life out…"
"I will have this place (looking around) tidied up…"

What else…?:

"The smoking: I'll be down to no more than five a-day…"

"Maybe, too, I'll have spoken to those in that help office, at the Regeneration Project…"

And what else…?:

"I can't see myself working yet, but maybe I'll have a few ideas…"

"And… I'll have sorted my head out more, so I won't need the drink to try and block it out…" "Doesn't work for long anyway…"

5. Scaling progress on the video of your life

Before scaling progress, it is helpful to make the following "link statement":

> "I'm wondering whether a little piece of what I have just described on the TV monitor is happening already. What might that be?"

Answer:

Then, scale progress:

> "On a scale of 1–10, where 10 stands for everything I have described on the screen happening as fully as possible, and 1 stands for it not having started, where am I right now on this scale?"

Answer (A majority of people answer 2–4.5):

Q: "How come I am at this number and not half a point lower?"

Answer:

Q: "What would I need to do to move half a point or 1 point further along, over, say, the next 2–3 weeks?"

Answer:

Q: "What will be good enough on this 1–10 scale for me? (Most people don't need to go for perfection at 10.)"

Answer:

6. What have you done or thought about that has been helpful to you so far?

(With any traumatic event or extreme situation in life, not only have we survived them, we have also done things that have helped us. Sometimes, we either forget or downplay these useful actions. It is helpful to remind ourselves of what we have done—and to do so often.)

I have done/thought about and found to be helpful, at least three things. They are

i.

ii.

iii.

Others (if applicable):

iv.

v.

Also:

7. What have you found helpful in what others have said or done?

(With some people, although they mean well, they are of little real help. Others—whether professionals, friends, family, etc.—are found to be helpful in things they do or say.)

List a few here:

a. Person's name:
   Helpful thing done/said:

b. Person's name:
   Helpful thing done/said:

c. Person's name:
   Helpful thing done/said:

d. Person's name:
    Helpful thing done/said:

8. The power of small steps

Sometimes, we can feel overwhelmed by what lies ahead and, as a result, do nothing to overcome the obstacles in our way. As mentioned in an earlier section, there is an old Chinese saying: "A journey of a thousand miles begins with a single step." What is mine? Can I think of one that is an *even smaller* step—one that I can take personally within the next 5–10 days?

"My first small step is…"

Now, answer the following:

"How and when will I take this small step?"

9. Who are your main encouragers and/or supporters?

It is important to bring to mind who your main supporters and encouragers are. It is even more important to write down their names, telephone numbers, and the ways they encourage, support, or nurture you. On low days, it is too easy to forget who they are and not ring or contact them. Writing their details below will help you stay connected.

a. Name:
    Mobile no.:
    Email address:

    How they encourage/support/nurture:

b. Name:
    Mobile no.:
    Email address:

    How they encourage/support/nurture:

c. Name:
    Mobile no.:
    Email address:

    How they encourage/support/nurture:

d. Name:
    Mobile no.:

Email address:

How they encourage/support/nurture:

e. Name:
    Mobile no.:
    Email address:

    How they encourage/support/nurture:

10. Write down your dream(s) for the future

This can help you visualise a realistic and achievable long-term future:

"What I would really like to do/achieve within the next few months/years is…"

(The importance of both visualising and writing out your dream(s) for the future is that you are more likely to achieve it (or them), or at least move a few small steps forward in that direction).

11. Those who have "done it", whom you admire most

Despite physical and/or psychological obstacles, many survivors of all sorts of things in life go on to live full and fulfilling lives. Reading their autobiographies can be both encouraging and inspiring. Simply bringing them to mind—and what they have managed to achieve and continue to achieve—is helpful.

Some of the more noteworthy in our current age are the following:

Bethany Hamilton

Bethany Hamilton (1990–present): After losing her arm in a shark attack at 13, she returned to professional surfing and became an inspiration for resilience and determination. Bethany Hamilton is an extraordinary individual whose story has inspired millions. She was born on February 8, 1990, in Lihue, Hawaii, growing up surrounded by the ocean. She began surfing at a very young age. By the time she was 13, she was already making waves in the competitive surfing world.

However, her life took a dramatic turn on October 31, 2003, when she was attacked by a 14-foot tiger shark while surfing off the coast of Kauai. The attack resulted in the loss of her left arm. Despite this life-altering event, Bethany's determination and faith remained unshaken.

Remarkably, she returned to surfing just one month later and adapted her technique to compete at the highest levels.

Bethany's resilience and achievements have made her a symbol of courage and perseverance. She has won numerous surfing competitions, written an autobiography titled Soul Surfer, and even had her story adapted into a feature film of the same name.

Beyond surfing, she is a motivational speaker, sharing her journey to inspire others to overcome challenges and pursue their dreams.

Today, Bethany continues to surf professionally, advocate for various causes, and embrace her roles as a wife and mother. Her unwavering spirit and positive outlook on life are truly remarkable. You can learn more about her journey on her official website: https:// bethanyhamilton.com/

Malala Yousafzai

Malala Yousafzai is a globally recognised advocate for girls' education and human rights. She was born on July 12, 1997, in Mingora, Swat Valley, Pakistan, growing up in a region where the Taliban imposed strict restrictions, including banning girls from attending school. Despite these challenges, Malala's passion for education was nurtured by her father, Ziauddin Yousafzai, who ran a school and supported her activism.

At the age of 11, Malala began writing a blog for the BBC under the pseudonym "Gul Makai," detailing her experiences and the challenges of living under Taliban rule. Her courage and determination made her a target, and on October 9, 2012, she was shot in the head by a Taliban gunman while riding a bus home from school. Miraculously, she survived and was treated at a hospital in Birmingham, UK.

Following her recovery, Malala became an international symbol of resilience and advocacy for education. In 2013, she co-founded the Malala Fund, which supports education initiatives worldwide. In 2014, she became the youngest-ever Nobel Peace Prize laureate at the age of 17, recognised for her efforts to promote education and equality.

Malala's journey has inspired millions, and she continues to work tirelessly to ensure that every child has access to education. Her autobiography, *I Am Malala*, provides a deeper insight into her life and mission. You can learn more about her remarkable story at NobelPrize.org.

Simon Weston[a]

He was a Welsh Guardsman who sustained 46 percent burns when the Royal Fleet Auxiliary ship HMS Sir Galahad

[a] Weston, S. Simon Weston CBE—Official Website. www.simonweston.com (accessed 22 May 2017).

was hit by an enemy missile in San Carlos Bay during the Falklands War in 1982.

He had years of reconstructive surgery, with 70 major operations or surgical procedures.

Simon tells his story to motivate and encourage those like him who want to move on to the next goal, whatever it may be. His message is one of single-minded determination, not only to accept what is but also to turn that to advantage. His career demonstrates clearly how a positive mental attitude can achieve great goals.

A key saying of Simon's that has encouraged many is this:

"The only obstacles to achieving one's targets and successes are those you create for yourself."

Some of Simon Weston's achievements:

- Set up 'The Weston Spirit', a liverpool-based young people's charity;
- Published four children's books;
- Set up a security business in South Wales;
- Awarded CBE for his charitable work

Frank Gardner[b]

He was BBC's Security Correspondent. In June 2004, while reporting from a suburb of Riyadh, Saudi Arabia, he was shot six times and seriously injured in an attack by al-Qaeda sympathisers. His cameraman colleague, Simon Cumbers, was shot dead in the attack. Being partly paralysed in his legs, Frank is now dependent on a wheelchair for life.

An Exeter University graduate, Frank Gardner's story hits close to home. He graduated with a degree in Arabic and Islamic Studies and later specialising in covering Middle Eastern conflicts post-War on Terror since the September 11 attacks in New York. He continues to be a role model for journalists and activists today.

Frank's achievements:

- Promoted to Major in the Royal Green Jackets Regiment of the British Army
- In the 2005 Birthday Honours, he was appointed officer of the Order of the British Empire (OBE)

[b] Gardner, Frank. (2017) Frank Gardner: BBC Security Correspondent, Journalist and Author. http://www.frankgardner.co.uk/ (accessed 22 May 2017); EXPOSÉ (2025) https://exepose.com/2025/02/22/frank-gardner-pioneering-journalist-in-activism-and-civil-rights-movements/

- Written two non-fiction books and a series of novels featuring the fictional SBS Officer-turned MI6 Operator, Nick Carlton

Nick Vujicic[c]

Nicholas James Vujicic (pronounced Voo-yee-cheech) was born in Melbourne, Australia, in 1982. His parents were Serbian Orthodox church immigrants from the former Yugoslavia. Having Tetra-Amelia syndrome, he was born without arms and legs. He had something that resembled a left foot at the base of his trunk, which he calls "my little chicken drumstick". Initially, his mother refused to see her newborn son when his condition was described to her, but later, as he grew up, she was one of his biggest supporters and encouragers.

In childhood, he struggled with depression and loneliness, questioning the purpose of life—whether he had a purpose at all. He was often bullied at school but remained determined to thrive. During his lowest times, he contemplated suicide and, at one point, made an unsuccessful attempt.

Nick refuses to allow his physical condition to limit his lifestyle. With his strong faith in God and the support

[c]Vujicic, N. (2017) Life Without Limbs. www.lifewithoutlimbs.org (accessed 22 May 2017); News Station 2 (2024) https://www.newsstation2.com/2024/09/06/a-minute-ago-nick-vujicic-passes-away-at-41-due-to-critical-health-condition/

of family and friends, has gone on to become a motivational speaker, musician, actor, and a prolific author. His first public-speaking engagement was when he was 19. He has spoken to schools, church groups, and business organisations.

Nick markets a motivational film for young people entitled *No arms, no legs, no worries!*

He has written seven books, titles of which include:

Life Without Limits: Inspiration of a Ridiculously Good Life (2010), *Your Life Without Limits* (2012), *and The Power of Unstoppable Faith* (2014).

(For the full list, see the Bibliography.)

Nick's hobbies include painting, fishing, and swimming. He is married with two sons and now lives in California, USA.

Nick Vujicic is a compelling example of how someone born with profound disabilities can go on to live a full and productive life, serving as an inspiration to others with less severe birth handicaps or disabilities resulting from injuries sustained in childhood or adulthood. Nick Vujicic passed on in 2024 age 41, due to a worsening critical health condition.

Kevin Hines[d]

Kevin Hines was born to drug-dealing parents and, after a chaotic early life, was taken into the foster care system. In 1986, he was adopted by Patrick and Debra Hines.

In his late teens, he developed extreme paranoia with delusions that people were out to kill him. In 1998, after a short period of mania, he was diagnosed with a bipolar condition with psychotic features.

Such was his increasing mental pain and anguish on 24 September 2000. Kevin looked online for ways to end his life. The Golden Gate Bridge in San Francisco, his hometown, was recommended by one dubious website. Since its construction in 1937, around 2,000 people have jumped to their deaths from the bridge (only 36, including Kevin, have survived).

While on the bus to the bridge, he was suddenly hit by ambivalence over his decision. Looking around at the other passengers, he sincerely believed that none of them cared whether he lived or died.

As with other survivors of suicide by jumping, a millisecond after his hands left the rail, he regretted it. He wanted an end to the mental pain, not to his life.

When he hit the water, he broke three spinal vertebrae. After fighting his way back up to the surface in the murky

[d] Hines, K. (2017) The Kevin Hines Story. www.kevinhinesstory.com (accessed 22 May 2017).

waters, he cried out continuously, "God, please save me!" and "I don't want to drown!" He was aware that all his depressive thoughts had disappeared. Miraculously, he was aware, too, that a sea lion had appeared and was gently supporting him from underneath. Kevin felt an overwhelming determination to survive. A coastguard speedboat rushed to his rescue, and they pulled him from the water.

After a series of operations, he was transferred to the mental ill-health wing of the hospital. He came to realise that "suicide should never be the answer", and that although some mental health issues can remain, life is the most powerful gift we have ever been given. He asserts that "rather than his cup being half full or half empty, his cup is overflowing and exuding positivity".

Kevin Hines is a filmmaker, motivational speaker, author, storyteller, and activist. As a survivor and now a thriver, he has devoted his life to spreading the message of living mentally healthy around the world. Kevin believes in the power of the human spirit and the fact that despite the problems we face, we can all find the ability to live mentally well. His mantra is this: "Life is a gift; that is why they call it the present. Cherish it always."

Kevin Hines serves on boards of various organisations championing mental health and has received many awards for his campaigning work. He is involved in policy work as an Ambassador to the US National Council for Behavioral Health.

In sharing his story, Kevin is fostering a critical bridge of hope between life and death for people caught in the pain of living with serious mental illness, difficult life circumstances, and more.

In 2006, he featured in the film *The Bridge*, produced by Eric Steed, and in 2013, he wrote the best-selling book *Cracked, not broken: Surviving and Thriving After a Suicide Attempt*. There are four YouTube videos about Kevin's amazing story of survival and now his work as a thriver. In one of these, he pleads with the general public to be on the lookout for strangers in emotional distress, suffering, and pain. He implores us to approach them— look them in the eyes—and ask, "Are you okay?" "Is there something wrong?" "Can we help?"

What people have said about Kevin Hines:

With an advanced degree of adversity, Kevin Hines survived the penultimate test to become uniquely qualified like no other, as an eloquent and effective witness for Wellness and Hope that an audience can ever hope to hear. He is more than a survivor; he is now a champion for anyone who needs to notch a win in the game of life.

Serni Solidarios, Director of Student Programmes/University of Puget Sound

I believe, with my whole heart, that Kevin's message saves lives.

Wende Nichols-Julien, Executive Director/ The California Conference for Equality and Justice

The entire world needs to hear Kevin's story.... He is able instantly, to connect to individuals in crisis…. His message is vital to any suicide prevention or resilience programme on the planet.

Commander Wayne-Boyd, US Marine Corps

I hope that you are aware of how much you have influenced my work. I tell your story quite often and even when I don't, you are more often than not, on my mind. You are saving lives, my friend, even more than you know, because you are influencing others out there who are saving lives too.

Captain Aaron Werbel PhD, Medical Services Corps, US Navy

Kevin's website[e] provides full information about his campaigning work.

Write down the names of others who have overcome incredible odds and are living their lives well (They do not have to be famous.)

a. Name:
    Achievements:

b. Name:
    Achievements:

c. Name:
    Achievements:

---

[e] One of the pages is devoted to merchandise, advertising tee shirts, and wrist bands with slogans, #HopeHelpsHeal, #KeepOnKeepingOn and #LifeIsAGift.

Sec. 6

12. What gives your life meaning and purpose?

"If we aim for nothing, we can be fairly certain we will hit it."

This statement is true both for those who have had traumatic life experiences and those who have not.

For those of us who experience pain or physical limitations, it is very important to put something into our lives that will give us a sense of meaning and purpose— something that will give it direction. This is the secret of good mental health, outlined in detail over 60 years ago by a psychotherapist Viktor Frankl (see the Bibliography).

For you to gain maximum benefit from this section, it is set out in three steps as follows:

a. "What I have done in the past that has given me a sense of meaning and purpose in my life?"

b. "What I am doing at present that gives me a sense of meaning and purpose in my life?"

c. "What will I do over the next few months to a year to give myself an increased sense of meaning and purpose in my life?"

… and my first small step will be:

By when:

13. Keeping all drugs at bay

Many survivors of severe trauma and stress are at risk of using drugs. It may be simply an increased use of nicotine or a heavier reliance on alcohol. It may take the form of over-the-counter drugs from the chemist and/or prescribed medications from a doctor. Nowadays, it is increasingly acknowledged that drugs for mental health issues are simply symptom-alleviation and *not* treatment. Some survivors say that using medication judiciously, can be helpful while practising self-help or being helped by others. Psychotherapists have highlighted this for many years; and more recently, psychiatrists are acknowledging this is the case (Ivanov and Schwartz, 2021). In a few circumstances, these drugs may be helpful to get survivors over a short-term difficulty. For commercial reasons, generally, the pharmaceutical companies that manufacture these drugs do not support short-term use. Neither are they interested in recommending withdrawal regimes, offering minimal advice only. However, the big psychopharma companies that manufacture psychotropic drugs have improved their withdrawal guidelines from "should be reduced over several weeks" to "should be withdrawn gradually to reduce the risk of discontinuation symptoms" (and similar) (BNF, 2025).

It is often seen as the easy option to increase drug intake as a way to soften the impact or provide some relief from painful memories and experiences we would rather forget. Although this may help a little in the short term, in the long run, *drugs do not work.*

Drug use—whether nicotine, alcohol, prescribed medication, or street drugs—can cause other problems in both the medium and long term. This can lead to serious life-threatening illnesses and premature death (see Gøtzsche, 2013).

We owe it to ourselves to educate ourselves and others about the harmful effects of all forms of drug use. Many health promotion and wellness organisations provide dozens of excellent leaflets and pamphlets, and these should be made as widely available as possible.

There has been a lot of discussion recently about antidepressants and their effects on the brain. What we know now is that most antidepressants only work in about 30 percent of cases after approximately 6 months. The idea of antidepressants "correcting a chemical imbalance in the brain" has been largely debunked (Griffin and Tyrrell, 2004; Moncrieff, 2022), and increased suicidal and homicidal tendencies and impotence are now widely reported side effects of several of them.

It is far better for our health if we empower ourselves and those we work with to take control by using methods involving the natural, God-given power of our mind and body. That is what this book is all about.

Here are some useful questions to ask yourself:

— How will I know when I am ready to have a conversation with my doctor about reducing my medication?
— As I begin to phase down my drug or alcohol use, what side effects will I notice becoming less frequent or less severe?
— When I am off all drugs, or reduce them to a more satisfactory level, how will that be helpful to me?
— Once I am clear of all drugs, what side effects will I notice are no longer present?

Other helpful questions:

What have I done so far to keep drinks and all drugs at bay?

What will I promise myself about keeping drinks and drugs at bay over the next year?

Breaking this down into small, realistic, and achievable steps, these are:

(1)

(2)

(3)

(4)

(5)

14. Seek out intimacy in relationships

Intimacy is a basic human need, with a spouse, family members, buddies, or close friends. This is not about sexual intimacy, but about closeness and connectedness with those who are near and dear to us. Some people prefer the companionship of a cat, a dog, or another type of pet. This is okay too.

As individuals, we feel more complete and fulfilled when intimacy plays an important part of our lives.

Helping survivors consider ways to achieve this can be both interesting and rewarding.

Reviewing our current intimate relationships can be a useful exercise.

Here are some questions to ask ourselves:

- How happy am I with my current level of intimate relationships?
- How could I become closer and more connected with them and/or others?

15. Reconnect with yourself

This form of reconnection can often be achieved by spending time alone, meditating, or making notes in a notebook or journal. It is about connecting deep within the very core of our being: our soul, our spirit.

We can review our thoughts about this—how it may have been useful to us in the past, and how it might have been working for us recently. Once we know what works or what helps, we will benefit by doing more of it.

16. Reconnect to a community

This again is a vital human need, unless we are self-declared loners or hermits.

Connection to an extended family, a neighbourhood, church, a community group, or an interest group, can be greatly beneficial. It holds even greater value to us when we contribute in some way. We feel accepted and appreciated by others—and, in turn, we appreciate them.

"Go national"

A man in his fifties who was an adult survivor of childhood abuse (mainly from his parents) decided to join a nationwide federation or community family trusts that promoted initiatives for strengthening marriage and the family. He helped support marriage preparation courses and parenting classes in his town.

17. Connect to God or "a higher power"

Most of us believe we are more than mind and body—that we have a spiritual aspect too, or there is a greater intelligence than ourselves or a being at work in life. Survivors with a religious faith can be encouraged to develop their spiritual connectedness through prayer, religious services, meditation, or study. They may seek conversion at this time. Throughout history, there have been many testimonies from people who have achieved great things through this form of connectedness. If you do not have this belief, the massive creativity and healing power of Nature itself may appeal.

18. Write a letter to someone you really admire

This exercise is a good one for survivors who need to "aim higher" with their expectations, both of themselves in the present and of what life might hold for them ahead.

The instructions are as follows:

1. Think of someone you really admire. This may be someone known to you (e.g. a boss, former head teacher, an inspiring friend or relation), or someone in the public arena.
2. Imagine you are going to write a letter to them, outlining all the things you admire about them.
3. Pick a quiet, private half hour, and actively write the letter (which, of course, will not be sent). Use a sheet of paper or a journal for this.

The effects of writing such an imaginary letter are:

- Recognition of qualities you would like to develop more in yourself
- Increased confidence and self-esteem
- A general boost in the "feel-good factor"

19. Kick the "PTSD" label into touch

Some professional colleagues seem to take great satisfaction in diagnosing survivors of severe trauma and stress with the label "PTSD". Labels like this, however, are generally not helpful and, for some, are seen as limiting at best and a life sentence at worst. Some professionals in years past were fond of such labels as "schizo-affective disorder", "chronic schizophrenia", and "manic-depressive psychosis". I have spent the latter part of my career helping survivors work on their symptoms to shed these labels and live purposeful and meaningful lives. Johnstone (2020) discusses the idea of symptoms having meaning in several contexts, particularly through her work on the Power Threat Meaning Framework (PTMF). There are meanings to be found behind emotional distress and psychological symptoms in the context of a person's life experiences. Our job as professionals or lay workers is to focus on understanding these meanings in the context of a person's life experiences.

A healthier and more positive way is to rename survivors' experiences as "post-traumatic growth" (PTG) or "post-traumatic success" (PTS) (see Bannink, 2014, 2016). These are both solution-focused terms and are more positive and helpful to survivors. Another is "post-traumatic stress reaction (PTSR)".

Diagnostic labels such as "disorder", "syndrome", and "disease" are medical terms, and in the field of mental health and emotional well-being, can be debilitating and a handicap to those who fully embrace them. It is often noted that survivors "with PTSD" simply exist, survivors with PTG, PTS, or PTSR go on to thrive!

20. The amazing effect of the first small step

Sometimes, we think about what we might like to do in the future and what we would like to achieve in life. Doubts and fears can get in the way of becoming the person we want to be.

The secret to making some headway in the right direction is to think what might be the first small step. Once you have done this, think of an *even smaller* step. Then *take it!*

21. Do not fall for the "depression" label

This is another diagnostic label often favoured by medical professionals and the pharmaceutical industry.

There are various definitions of depression, and these can vary from practitioner to practitioner.

Currently, my two preferred definitions are those described by Griffin:

"Unexpressed (negative) emotion"; and/or

"Undeclared or unresolved issues from the past"

(Griffin, 2004)

Neuroscience now supports the view that the traditional biochemical definition of depression—that the brain has a chemical imbalance—is, at best, a half-truth or, at worst, false. In her 2022 research papers, Professor Joanna Moncrieff (Moncrieff, J., 2022 and Moncrieff, J., 2022a) debunked the serotonin deficit theory of depression.

Other helpful techniques/questions to promote Thriving:

22. What helped you survive at the time of the incident?

23. **What else helped?**

24. **What strengths and skills did you bring into play at the time?**

25. **What else have you been through in life that was difficult, and what helped you then?**

26. **Which of the things that helped you then could be useful to you again now?**

27. **Thinking of others who have gone through the same or a similar ordeal, what helped that person/those people deal with it?**

28. **What does it mean to you to have survived these traumatic events?**

29. **When these traumatic events are even less of a problem in your life, what will you be thinking about and doing instead?**

30. How have the experiences and events you have gone through made you a stronger person?

31. How have the experiences and events you have gone through made you a more determined person?

32. How do you maintain your hope that you can regain an even better life in the future?

33. How will others close to you know how well you have succeeded in living life to the full?

34. What helps you most in keeping any intrusive thoughts and memories under control?

35. Which experiences of safety or comfort from the past do you make use of now?

36. What symbol of safety or comfort from the past do /could you make use of now?

37. What rituals could you perform when you have reached your goal of living life to the full? How would you celebrate?

38. In spite of all that has happened, how do you remain hopeful and optimistic about the future?

39. If you need more hope, how would you make that happen?

A growing number of survivors of severe trauma can testify to the effectiveness of the tools and techniques shared in this book in treating both depression and "the lows". These outcomes are achieved without the use of medication, or, at most, having it prescribed in the short term only.

Finally, in conclusion, the "thriving" state not only promotes healthy lives, but also promotes longer and more productive lives. Over the 20- plus years of teaching 2-day workshops on this subject (see Appendix H), I have had the privilege of meeting many fellow thrivers who have since become therapists. Below are some of their testimonies (I have anonymised all names to protect their privacy, although I know many would not mind):

"Coming through what I experienced, to a point now where I cannot believe how full and meaningful

Sec. 6

my life is, I just want to give back to others so they can fully live, too."

Sandra, Manchester, UK

"Although I will never forget the death and carnage I witnessed, I know now that I need not be affected by it as I was for a while, following the incident. With my tried and tested techniques for triggers and unwanted thoughts, I feel equipped to deal with any reminders or memories from that terrible time. Now, I am living my life more fully and enjoyably than I ever did before it happened. In some way, I'm grateful for the incident for how I'm living now. Does that sound weird?"

Brian, Perth, Western Australia

"I lost my son in a tragic set of circumstances and for which I blamed myself. I felt suicidal, only in the sense I would be reunited with him in death. I went through a two-year nightmare and had to go away to a healing retreat. While there, I was taught some surprisingly helpful techniques and at the same time was encouraged to read Gerald L. Sittser's book, *A Grace Disguised: How the Soul Grows Through Loss.* Sittser lost most of his family in a tragic car crash, yet he was still able to forgive and go on to live life to the full. I thought to myself: "I will, can, and must do that, too". I am now a qualified therapist helping other survivors along their journey to the thriving life."

Lee Wong, Singapore

Reassuring Things for Survivors to Know

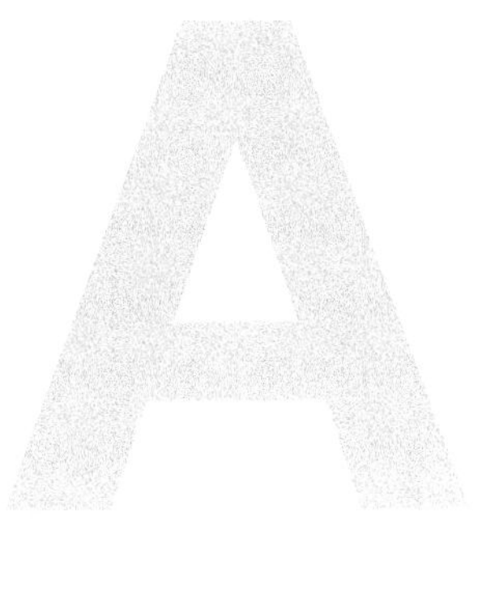

1. Only about 15% of people who experience a traumatic incident will develop symptoms that last more than a few weeks.
2. There are both positive and negative effects from severe trauma and stress experiences.
3. If you experience symptoms, you do not necessarily need to seek therapy from a professional or field expert. Self-help and "buddy-aid" are sufficient in many cases.
4. Getting professional help does not mean you are weak. It takes great courage to meet, in confidence, with a complete stranger to talk through your experiences.

5. Whatever traumatic event you have experienced, when meeting with a professional, you do not have to recount everything or remember all that happened. Meeting up with a professional does not mean you are going mad and/or out of control.

6. Symptoms can be dealt with simply and effectively in the short term—without the use of medication, "depth psychology", or long-term psychotherapy. (In some extreme cases, a short course of medication may be helpful.)

7. Buying into "a PTSD diagnosis", with its long-term implications, is generally unhelpful.

8. An achievable and realistic aim in recovery is a happier, more fulfilling, meaningful, peaceful, and joyous life.

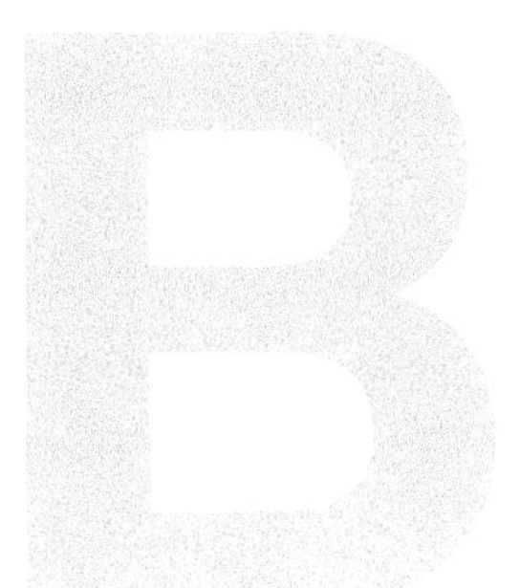

What Survivors Have Found to be Helpful in This Work

Survivors found it helpful when people:

- Enabled identification of conflicts they were experiencing or feeling.
- Encouraged working through these issues—if that was what they wanted.
- Promoted self-esteem and self-confidence.
- Encouraged them to take control of their lives.
- Allowed them to choose the goals of therapy following their wishes and values.
- Maximised collaboration, minimised resistance in the work.
- Encouraged them to give up secrecy and shame in their lives.

- Gave information—both verbal and written.
- Provided a good quality therapeutic relationship for disclosing. This mobilised the person's capacity for self-healing and growth.
- Built a trusting relationship.
- Provided acceptance, and supported and encouraged them to confront conflicts where appropriate.
- Helped them to share thoughts and feelings.
- Showed understanding.
- Gave time.
- Enabled correct apportionment of blame.
- Acknowledged, validated, and normalised their thoughts and feelings wherever possible.
- Helped them to express emotions, thoughts, and feelings.
- Simply allowed them to disclose or divulge what happened in their way and at their own pace.
- Asked what they were seeking in treatment and how they would know when their treatment is successful.
- Did not assume that they needed to go back and work through traumatic memories. (Some do, some do not.)
- On rare occasions, made provisions (e.g. contracts) for safety from suicide, homicide, and other potentially dangerous situations when necessary. These worked best when they were mutual.

- Remained focused on the goals of treatment rather than getting lost in the gory details.
- Avoided giving the message that the person is "damaged goods" or that their future is determined by the traumatic or stressful incident they experienced.
- Admitted sometimes to getting it wrong.
- Enabled them to feel safe.

Helpful Questions and Statements from the Welfare Worker

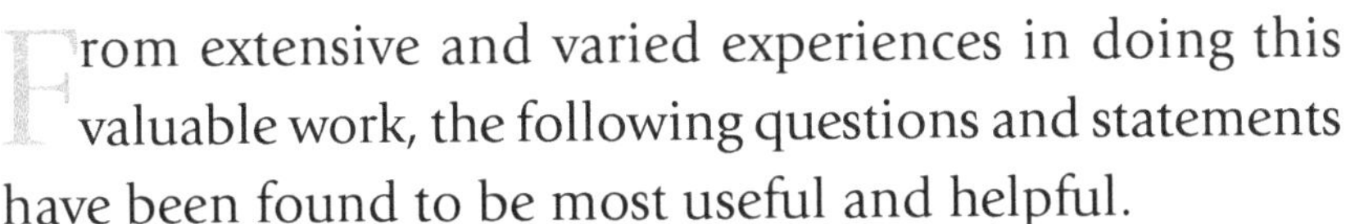

From extensive and varied experiences in doing this valuable work, the following questions and statements have been found to be most useful and helpful.

1. "How would you like to use these sessions?"
2. "What do you think your friends, boss, or others might begin to notice about you as you sort things out in your own mind and continue to move forward?"
3. "What strengths, qualities, or special abilities did you call into play to survive that time or those incidents?"

4. "What have you done so far, not only to sort things out in your own mind, but also to be live your life well?"

5. "How much detail do you need to tell me before you are ready to move on?"

6. "What do you feel you need to tell me so I can be most helpful to you?"

7. "What particular techniques do you use to counteract any unwelcome thoughts you might be having?"

8. "On a scale of 1–10, where are you now in terms of living your life well?"

9. "What we know from this type of work is that people can work through the things that might be holding them back."

10. "It is quite common for people to feel guilty about what happened."

11. "What has been particularly helpful to you so far in expressing your anger in safe ways?"

12. "What particular strengths, qualities, or resources do you have that have been helpful to you in the past, and which could be useful to you in the months and years to come?"

13. "What would be the first (smallest) sign that things are getting better, that this incident is having less of an impact on your life?"

14. "What will you be doing differently when this (incident) becomes less of a problem in your life?"

15. "What will you be doing differently with your time?"

16. "What useful things will you be in the habit of saying to yourself?"

17. "What will you be thinking about (or doing) *instead* of thinking about the past?"

18. "Tell me about times when some of these are already happening, even to a small extent."

19. "What difference do you think these healing changes will make once they have been present in your life for a long period—weeks, days, months, or even years?"

20. "What do you think your (significant other) would say is the first sign that things are getting better? What do you think they would notice first?"

21. "What other difficulties have you been through, and what helped you then?"

22. "Which of those things that helped you then could be useful to you again now?"

23. "What does surviving these traumatic events mean to you?"

24. "What difference do the changes you have accomplished make to your family now, and for future generations?"

25. "What helpful symbol of safety or comfort from the past could you use for the work you are doing here?"
26. "When you have reached the thriver stage, what ritual would you like to use to celebrate?"

(I am grateful to Fredrike Bannink for granting permission to include in this list some additional questions from her highly recommended book, *1001 Solution Focused Questions*, published by W.W. Norton & Company.)

The Three Stages: Victim–Survivor–Thriver (Living Life to the Full, or as Full as Possible)

Information for survivors about the characteristics of each stage:

Victim

- This is the first stage of healing. First, it is important for you to face the reality of the bad or unfortunate thing that happened.
- You can then acknowledge the negative feelings and emotions that might be around (grief, anger,

sadness, disappointment, frustration, despair, hopelessness, helplessness, etc.).

- Allow yourself to experience these feelings and emotions—and to express them.
- This is a vital part of healing, plus a valuable part of this stage.
- It is also important to recognise that what happened was *not your fault*, so you can let go of self-blame and shame. (In the rare cases where it was partly your fault, it is important to attribute only the correct proportion of blame to yourself. Then, consider in what ways, constructively, you may make amends for what occurred.)
- Find the courage to tell someone else what happened to you; this breaks down the isolation.
- As soon as the victim stage has been acknowledged and understood, you can move into the next stage—*Survivor*.

Survivor

- This begins when you understand you have lived beyond the traumatic or highly stressful experience/s that occurred.
- This stage reinforces the fact that it happened in the past.

- Then questions may be asked: "How did I survive it?", "How did I do it?", and "What strengths and resources did I use?"
- Acknowledgment of survivorhood involves:
  - Developing an inventory of positive personality characteristics.
  - Identifying and appreciating the internal strengths (knowledge, courage, spirituality, and other positive aspects of self) that have brought you this far.
  - Identifying external resources (friends, support groups, telephone helplines, supportive family members, community support, etc.) at the time of the incident/s and afterwards.
- At this stage, you will regain the ability to function in everyday life—work, family time, household chores, time with friends, hobbies, community activities, and more.
- Once you have acknowledged that you have survived—with the skills, strengths, qualities, and resources that have carried you through to survival and eventual wellbeing—move on to thriving, living life to the full, and living a purposeful and meaningful life as possible.

Thriver—Living Life to the Full

- This allows you more freedom than in the earlier stages.
- It allows you to experience a more compelling present and contemplate a more vivid and fulfilling future than your past.
- It is now possible to enjoy life to the fullest, regardless of the physical limitations you may have.
- It is worthwhile to explore the possibilities and dreams for the future that you may be envisioning right now.
- It is now possible for you to express yourself in the most personally rewarding and creative ways available to you.
- In this stage, your current experiences and relationships may increasingly evoke a sense of immediacy, wonder, and an enhanced potential for future growth.
- You have a clear idea now about what gives you meaning and purpose in life.
- You are able to clearly state your goals for the future.
- You are living life to the full. Good feelings about both yourself and your world abound like never before.

(The above points have been developed from ideas outlined by Yvonne Dolan in her book, *Beyond Survival: Living Well is the Best Revenge*, BT Press, 2000.)

The 5 o'clock Rule (for the First Sessions)

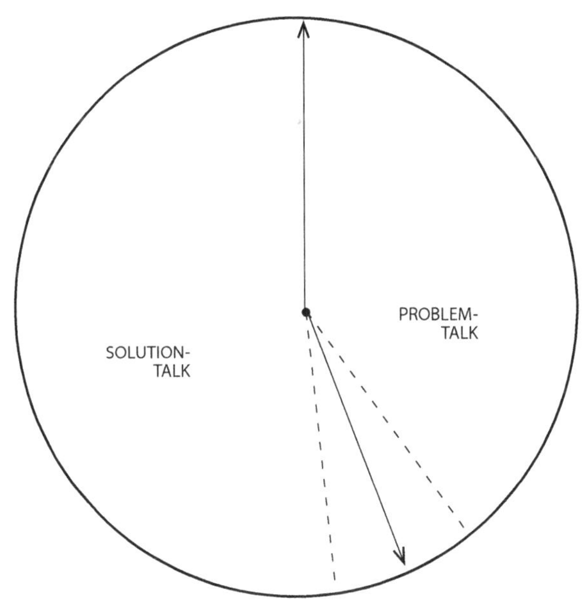

Notes:

1. 'Solution-talk' consists of things like problem-free talk, strengths-based questions, exceptions, pre-session change, the miracle question, scaling, and identification of small steps.

2. 'Problem-talk' consists of what the nature of the problem is: its effects on the client's life, signs and symptoms, negativity, general difficulties, failed solutions, setbacks, etc.

3. The two sections in the diagram are simply overall proportions of the 60 minutes. It does not mean that the first 25 minutes consists only of 'problem-talk' (the session may begin with a problem-free talk). Also, as the client is outlining their problem story, the worker will be interrupting with strengths-based questions and asking for exceptions.

4. The 25 minutes of problem-talk is only a guide. It may lessened (as in the diagram). It may also be slightly more, but ideally, still less than 30 minutes; otherwise, the client would be trained the wrong way.

Blocks to Disclosing

Below is a comprehensive list of the main "blocks" that survivors may have when speaking to a professional worker. With some of these, the survivor simply will not come forward at all. Many who do may struggle to speak openly because one or several of these blocks get in the way. If you can identify the block(s) together with the survivor, you may be able to help them move forward.

In some cases, survivors can be helped therapeutically without needing to disclose what happened.

Worker's gender

Fear of rejection

Shame

Unable to articulate

Not being believed

Non-recognition

Loss of control

Special needs disability

Feeling unsafe

Embarrassment

Religious beliefs

Fear of being judged

Fear of being seen as
weak/soft/not able
to cope

Fear of consequences

Fear of someone important
finding out

Lack of trust

Worker is perceived as not
understanding

Unsure reaction of the
worker

Betrayal of family/others

Worker's inexperience

Concerns about official
secrets

Guilt

Denial

Worker's rank/perceived
status

Feeling "contaminated" by the abuse/incident and therefore not wanting to "infect" or affect the worker

Not wanting to be seen in a poor light by the worker

Having been told by the perpetrator or others to remain silent

Previous poor experiences when disclosing

Not trusting the environment (answer phone for messages, paper-thin walls, too many windows, and so on)

Believing the worker's knowledge of the subject is insufficient

Worker is lacking empathy

How to Avoid Retraumatisation and Revictimisation

The following eight tips have proven invaluable in helping workers do this important work successfully and in a way that is truly helpful for survivors.

1. Show compassion and deep empathy.
2. As the survivor discloses: acknowledge, validate, and normalise all feelings and sensations expressed.
3. Ask strength-based questions—interjecting, when appropriate—while the survivor is disclosing, as follows:
   - How did you cope at the time?
     - What got you through all this?
     - What helped the most?
     - How did you do that?
     - How did you know how to do that?

- Looking back on what happened, in what ways has it made you a more determined and/or stronger person?
- Although it was awful, which aspects of surviving it have helped make you a better person?

4. It is important to sincerely compliment the survivor where appropriate, both during their moment of disclosure, and most importantly, at the end of the session.
5. Treat the details of the disclosure with care, respect, and in a supportive manner.
6. Value and affirm the survivor, verbally and non-verbally.
7. Keep both your own and your survivor's eyes on the treatment goals.
8. Adhere to the "5 o'clock rule" (see Henden, 2017).

Benefits of Doing This Important Work

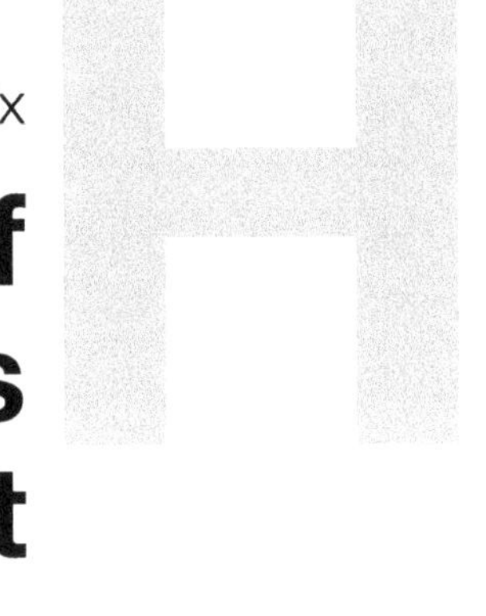

Whether you are a survivor or a practitioner reading this appendix, the comprehensive list on the right-hand side outlines the countless benefits to be gained from engaging in this important work.

If you are a survivor: what is stopping you? What is your next small step?

No to:	Yes to:
Life of fear and anxiety	Successful personal relationships
Marital/couple break-up	Quality family life
Existence as a victim/survivor	Passing on tips and techniques to other survivors

No to:	Yes to:
Constant pulling around "the PTSD ball and chain"	Living life well
Excessive use of drinks, drugs, or tobacco for coping	Healthy living/eating
Feeling out of control	Feeling in control; living life well
Finding difficulty resting or doing nothing in particular	Physical fitness as much as possible
Feelings of being stuck	Feelings of great joy from time to time
Fearful of unexpected triggers	Welcoming triggers to practise techniques learned
Difficulties with everyday functioning	Getting on well with day-to-day tasks
Feeling that life is meaningless and pointless	Having a sense of meaning and purpose in life
Disturbed sleep with recurrent nightmares	Settled sleep patterns
Feeling odd and disconnected from people	Enjoying connectedness with people—especially loved ones

No to:	Yes to:
Constantly reliving what happened	Regarding what happened as being part of life, but not being dominated by it
General unhappiness and discontent with life	Personal goals and targets in life to look forward to
Sudden and unpredictable outbursts of anger	Safely controlled aggression
Excessively isolating self from family and friends, in particular	Having a forward view of life, in terms of chapters yet to be written

Two-Day Solution-Focused Workshops on Working with Severe Trauma and Stress

These 2-day workshops have been running for over 25 years, dealing with both severe adult trauma and stress and adult survivors of child abuse and neglect.

For enquiries, please email john@ johnhendenconsultancy.co.uk

The workshop content and learning objectives are outlined below:

Workshop Content

- Welcome and Introductions
- Contracting around making it safe for people to work

- Aims and objectives
- Outline plan for the 2 days
- The Solution-Focused approach
- Scaling confidence
- Naming the trauma: road traffic crashes, armed robbery, sudden death, muggings, near-death experiences, natural disasters, terrorist attacks, rape, child abuse and neglect, and threats to kill
- What has been found to have worked in one-on-one work with survivors
- What survivors have found helpful
- The three stages: "victim", "survivor", and "thriver"
- The 25 basic tools and techniques of solution-focused therapy
- Survival skills outlined
- Dealing with anger and "the solution-focused feelings tank"
- Applying basic solution-focused techniques to survivors
- Sticking to "the 5 o'clock rule"
- Disclosing/divulging what happened
- The detail: how much is necessary to know?
- Blocks to disclosing
- What equips us to do this work?
- Introducing specialised techniques

- Implications of this type of work for workers and how they can look after themselves
- Getting to know the "thriver" stage
- The specialised techniques:
  - "Let it go…Let it go…let it go"
  - The "Stop!" technique and "replaying the video" later
  - "That was then, this is now"
  - "Dual awareness" for dealing with intrusive thoughts
  - The rainy-day letter
  - Letter from the future plus how to use it
  - "Park it…and move on"
  - The solution-focused feelings tank
  - Fast-forwarding the video of your life
  - Write, read, and shred/burn
  - "Shrinking" for dealing with flashbacks of incoming missiles
  - Dealing with "the lows"
- Purpose and meaning in life/Living life as full as possible
- Improving our practice from today
- Workshop roundup/summary
- Recommended reading list
- Workshop evaluation

Learning Outcomes

At the end of the workshop, attendees will be able to:

- Demonstrate an increased understanding of severe trauma and stress and the effects of child abuse and neglect
- Describe the characteristics of the "victimhood", "survivorhood", and "thriverhood" ("living life well"/as full as possible)
- Describe the basic solution-focused tools and techniques used with survivors
- Use a variety of specialised tools and techniques for helping survivors move further towards *thriverhood*/ living life well/their authentic self
- Recognise how these specialised techniques can be applied to other types of potentially traumatic situations
- List the main points survivors have made about how practitioners can best be helpful
- Name the pitfalls when working with survivors of severe trauma and stress
- Highlight the most helpful and useful questions to ask

- List the key ways practitioners can look after themselves to enable them to undertake this important work
- Feel more confident in their work with a wide range of survivors

Supporting Research Evidence for Solution-Focused Brief Therapy

Still, the main text showing the evidence base for solution-focused therapy (SFT) is:

Franklin, C., Trepper, TS, Gingerich, W. J., & McCollum, E.E. (2012) Solution-Focused Brief Therapy: a handbook of evidence-based practice. OUP

A Solution-Focused Therapy Evaluation List

This used to be hosted and maintained by Emeritus Consultant Psychiatrist Dr. Alasdair Macdonald. However, due to the closure of his website, this is no longer available.

15 June 2016 Update
One of the last abbreviated updates before the closure of the site is as follows:

(Reproduced in part with thanks and full acknowledgement to Dr. Macdonald)

More than 2,300 publications are produced annually. Currently, there are 8 meta-analyses, 6 systematic reviews, 245 relevant outcome studies, including 100 randomised controlled trials showing the benefits from solution-focused approaches, with 69 showing benefits over existing treatments. Of 73 comparison studies, 57 favour solution-focused therapy (SFT). Effectiveness data are also available from over 8,000 cases with a success rate exceeding 60%, requiring an average of 3 to 6.5 sessions of therapy time.

The National Registry of Evidence-based Programs and Practices (NREPP) is approved by the US Federal Government: www.samhsa.gov; SAMHSA. The State of Washington, State of Oregon (www.oregon.gov/DHS), and State of Texas are examining evidence. Minnesota, Michigan, and California have organisations using SFT. Finland has a master's degree program in SFT, and Singapore has an approved accreditation programme.

Canada has a registration body for practitioners and therapists. Sweden, Poland, Germany, and Austria recognise it within their systemic practice qualification. Wales (UK) includes it in their primary mental health programme.

Many recent publications were in Farsi, Finnish, French, German, Korean, and Turkish. By 2014, there were 180 publications in Mandarin (including 60 from Taiwan) as against 45 in 2009. So, this evaluation list confirms the value of the model, but is no longer sufficient in itself.

Meta-analyses (only a few studies listed here)

Carr A., Hartnett D., Brosnan E., Sharry J. (2016). Parents Plus systemic, solution-focused parent training programs: Description, review of the evidence-base, and meta-analysis. Family Process. Parents Plus (PP) programs are systemic, solution-focused, group-based interventions designed both as preventive interventions and as treatment programs for families with child-focused problems.

Each program typically consists of 6–9 group sessions with 8–12 participants. A group session is for 2 hours; programs span 2–3 months. With 17 studies: 919 parents engaged in PP training and 440 were in the waiting list control (WLC) or treatment as usual (TAU) control groups.

With six randomised controlled trials (RCTs), six non-RCTs, and with five uncontrolled single group outcome studies. Dropout rates before post-treatment assessment (range: 2%–33%). Meta-analysis of ten controlled studies: effect size 0.58. Pooled effect sizes: child behaviour problems: PP clients better than approximately 73% of controls; goal attainment: PP clients better than 94% of controls; parental satisfaction: PP clients better than 80% of controls; parental stress: PP clients better than 70% of controls. "In most studies, follow-up assessments showed that gains were maintained several months later." (alan.carr@ucd.ie)

Kim J. S. (2008). Examining the effectiveness of solution-focused brief therapy: A meta-analysis. Research on Social Work Practice 18:107–116. 22 studies; many factors examined. Small effects in favour of SFT; best for personal behaviour change, effect size estimate 26 (sig. $p<0.05$). Thus, SFT is equivalent to other therapies. (Dissertation: Examining the Effectiveness of Solution-focused Brief Therapy: A Meta-Analysis Using Random Effects Modelling. University of Michigan database. Up to 6.5 sessions required. Competence in SFT requires >20 hours of training) (johnny.kim@du.edu)

Park Jung-im (2014). Meta-analysis of the effect of the solution-focused group counseling program for elementary school students. Journal of the Korea Contents Association

14(11): 476–485. URL: http://www.dbpia. co.kr/ Article/3535871. Master's theses, doctoral dissertations, and journal articles published in Korea up to May 2014 were systematically reviewed. A total of 20 studies were eligible for the inclusion criteria. The mean effect sizes and test for homogeneity of effect size (Q-statistic) were analysed using the Comprehensive Meta-Analysis software2.0. Main findings: average effect sizes for Solution-Focused Group Counseling Program were ES 1.61 in self-esteem, ES 1.35 in school adjustment capacity, ES 1.07 in interpersonal relationship, and ES 1.03 in self-efficacy. Moderating variables were focused on self-esteem and sessions of 1 hour.

Gong H., Hsu W. S. (2015). A meta-analysis on the effectiveness of solution-focused brief therapy: evidences from mainland and Taiwan. Studies of Psychology and Behaviors (CSSCI) 13(6): 709–803. With 33 studies, totalling 1,147 participants. With 33 studies from Taiwan and China: 1,147 participants. Overall effect size, 0.99; school, 1.01; medical settings, 0.94; mainland, 1.03; and Taiwan, 0.92. Overall, 1.07 at follow-up. No correlation with the year of publication. Effective for different kinds of problems and improves client's ability to solve problems by themselves. (weisuhsu@ ntnu.edu.tw) (Mandarin)

Systematic reviews (only a few studies listed here)

Bond C., Woods K., Humphrey N., Symes W., Green L. (2013). The effectiveness of solution focused brief therapy with children and families: a systematic and critical evaluation of the literature from 1990–2010. Journal of Child Psychology and Psychiatry doi: 10.1111/jcpp.12058.

With 38 studies included: nine applied SFBT to internalising child behaviour problems; three applied SFBT to both internalising and externalising child behaviour problems; 15 applied the approach to externalising child behaviour problems, and 9 evaluated the application of SFBT in relation to a range of other issues. Provides tentative support for the use of SFBT; particularly effective as an early intervention when presenting problems are not severe.

Gingerich W. J., Peterson L. T. (2013). Effectiveness of Solution-Focused Brief Therapy: A Systematic Qualitative Review of Controlled Outcome Studies. Research on Social Work Practice 23(3): 266–283. All available controlled outcome studies of SFBT: 43 studies were abstracted: 32 (74%) of the studies reported significant positive benefit from SFBT; and 10 (23%) reported positive trends. The strongest evidence of effectiveness came in the treatment of depression in adults where four separate studies found SFBT to be comparable to well-established alternative treatments. Three studies examined the length of treatment and all found that SFBT used fewer sessions than alternative therapies. The studies reviewed provide strong evidence that SFBT is an effective treatment for a wide variety of behavioural and psychological outcomes, and it may be briefer—and therefore less costly—than alternative approaches. (http://rsw.sagepub. com/content/ early/2013/01/22/1049731512470859) DOI: 10.1177/1049731512470859

Lovelock H., Matthews R., Murphy K. (2011). Evidence-based psychological interventions in the treatment of mental disorders: a literature review. Australian Psychological Association http://www.psychology.org.au/ Assets/Files/ Evidence-Based-Psychological-Interventions. pdf. SFBT shows Level II effectiveness for depression, anxiety, and substance misuse.

Published follow-up studies (245): randomised controlled studies (100) (only a few studies listed here)

Ahramian A., Ahmadi A., Shamseddinilory S., Yousefi S., Abdolahi S., Soudani M., Ghazi G. (2014). The effectiveness of group training of solution-focused approach on marriage adjustment of couples that call on Bushehr family counseling centers. (Iran) Terapevticheskii Arkhiv

86(1s). Couples; randomised; 22 experiments (exp.) for solution-focused (SF) groups/22 controls. Exp. results: significant improvement in marital adjustment. (Persian)

Baldry E., Bratel J., Dunsire M., Durrant M. (2005). Keeping Children with a Disability Safely in their Families. Practice: Social Work in Action 17(3):143–156. DOI:10.1080/09503150500285099 With 55 caregivers from 40 families in crisis; family-centred intervention programmes (Australia). Objective measures: empowerment, emotional support, parent–child involvement, abuse potential, family functioning, symptom reduction, hope, happiness, and worker–client alliance; also, qualitative interviews. Significant improvement in abuse potential and emotional support at 6 months and 12 months ($p < 0.001$). Symptom reduction and emotional support predicted 86% of the variance at 12 months. Helpful: wholly attentive listening, support, increased parent control/empowerment, validation, and maintaining a strengths focus; programmes being family-focused, having 24 hours/phone availability, being home-based, with small case-loads, financial support, and worker consistency. (e.baldry@unsw.edu.au)

Bagajan K. Q., Khanahmadi O., Chaharborj Z. M., Chenaparchi M. (2016). The Impact of Solution-Focused Brief Therapy on the Improvement of the Psychological Wellbeing of Family Supervisor Women. International

Journal of Social, Behavioral, Educational, Economic, Business and Industrial Engineering 10 (1). Random: 15 exp. with 5 SF sessions/15 controls no treatment. Significant increase in well-being for exp. at post-test. (kawe.ghaderi@ gmail.com) (Persian)

Grant A. M. (2012). Making Positive Change: A Randomized Study Comparing Solution-Focused vs. Problem-Focused Coaching Questions. J Systemic Therapies 31(2): 21–35. Random: real problem and set goal. Measures: positive and negative affect, self-efficacy, goal attainment. With 108 participants: problem-focused coaching questions; 117 participants: solution-focused questions including future-oriented question; then, a second set of measures. Both effective in enhancing goal approach; solution-focused group significantly greater increases in goal approach, positive affect, decreased negative affect, and increased self-efficacy; and generated significantly more action steps to help them reach their goal. Although real-life coaching conversations are not solely solution-focused or solely problem-focused, agents of change should aim for a solution-focused theme.

Hsu W. S., Chen Y. F., Sun S. T. M., Wu C. Y., Cheng H. C. (2009). A study of working alliance, counselor's effectiveness, and client's satisfaction of solution-focused real-time web counseling on Taiwanese college students. Bulletin of Southern Taiwan University 34 (2), 57–70.

Real-time web counselling designed by Information Management of National Chi Nan University, Taiwan. Three counsellors trained. Randomised: 8 students SF; 10 students non-sf; 1–6 weekly sessions. Pre-post measures: better scores for alliance and effectiveness after the first session for SF. Exp. group with significantly higher scores for counsellor effectiveness and client satisfaction, not alliance. (weisuhsu@ ntnu.edu.tw)

Lindforss L., Magnusson D. (1997). Solution-focused therapy in prison. Contemporary Family Therapy 19:89–104. With two randomised studies: (1) Pilot study 14/21 (66%) exp. and 19/21 (90%) controls reoffended at 20 months. (2) With 30 exp.; 29 controls; 16-month follow-up. With 18 (60%) reoffend in exp., 25 (86%) in control; more drug offences and more total offences in controls. With an average of five sessions; 2.7 million Swedish crowns saved by reduced reoffending. (lindforss@ chello.se; dan.magnusson@brottsforebygganderadet.se)

Ma Jianmin (2015). Focus-solving model used in patients with chronic health. Education Management Journal of Clinical Nursing 4. Doi: 10.3969/j.issn.1671-8933.2015.04.017 Chronic hepatitis B; random: 50 exp. SF health education/50 controls routine education. Knowledge significantly increased post-test; liver function improved. (Mandarin)

SunYunxia, Wu Lin, Guo Xiangrong (2015). Application effects of solution focused approach on psychological nursing in patients with MRI examination Chinese Journal of Modern Nursing 26. MRI subjects with claustrophobia; random; 64 exp. with five sessions of SF counselling/64 TAU. Patients and caregivers report less anxiety/depression/dyspnea 26.5% exp. vs. 37.5%/sweating 46.8% vs. 64.1%: p <0.05. doi: 10.3760/cma.j.issn.1674-2907.2015.26.005 (Mandarin)

Theeboom T., Beersma B., Van Vianen A. E. M. (2015). The differential effects of solution-focused and problem-focused coaching questions on the affect, attentional control and cognitive flexibility of undergraduate students experiencing study-related stress. Journal of Positive Psychology, DOI: 10.1080/17439760.2015.111712661. Random: 31 exp. SF questions about preferred future/30 controls problem-focused questions; higher positive affect, lower negative affect in exp.; no effect on attentional control. Repeat: 28 exp./26 controls: same results for affect. More cognitive flexibility in exp.; apparently not mediated by positive affect. (t.theeboom@uva.nl)

Wang Shan, Xu Jin-zhi, Zhang Jin-feng (2015). Effects of solution-focused approach in the rehabilitation training of patients with lung cancer. Chinese Journal of General Practice 13(10). Random: 40 exp. rehab exercises;

SFT/40 controls rehab exercises. Quality of life and health status significantly better ($p < 0.05$) in exp. at 3 months. (Mandarin)

Zhou Li-li, Ji Tian-rong, Liu Feng, Bu Zhi-hua, Liu Li, Yang Xiao-yun (2013). Effect of nursing intervention based on solution-focused approach on self-management ability of patients with maintenance hemodialysis. Chinese Journal of Modern Nursing 34. Randomised: 60 exp. (SF nursing)/60 controls (routine nursing). With a 6-month follow-up: knowledge of disease and self-management significantly improved in exp. group. Doi:10.3760/cma.j. issn.1674-2907.2013.34.004 (Mandarin)

Comparison studies (73) (only a few studies listed here)

Amiri H., Sharme M. S., Zarchi A. K., Bahari F., Binesh A. (2013). Effectiveness of Solution-Focused Communication Training (SFCT) in Nurses' Communication Skills. Iranian Journal of Military Medicine 14 (4): 279–286. With 71 nurses from medical–surgical departments of Tehran hospital. With an 8-hour workshop; pre-test; post-test 2 months after. With three questionnaires completed (participant, head nurse, colleagues). Mean difference statistically significant [$p = 0/001$]; also between mean scores of 4 subscales of nurses' communication skills. (amirizh@yahoo.com)

Antle B. F., Barbee A. P., Christensen D. N., Martin M. H. (2008). Solution-based casework in child welfare: preliminary evaluation research. Journal of Public Health Child Welfare 2(2): 197–227. Study 1: fully trained workers, 27 cases; minimally trained, 21 cases. Better compliance, fewer legal actions, and fewer removals in the trained group. Study 2: 51 cases from fully trained, 49 minimally trained. Better compliance and goal achievement in both urban and rural areas.

Connell M. A. (2014). Modifying Academic Performance Using Online Grade Book Review During Solution-Focused Brief Therapy. Walden University Dissertation 3631272. Three groups of at-risk students: Group 1 SFBT only (18); Group 2 (20) SFBT and Online Grade Book Review (JumpRope); and Group 3 (22) JumpRope alone. Results suggested statistical significance of including gradebook review within SFBT resulted in improved academic performance.

Corcoran J. A. (2006). A comparison group study of solution-focused therapy versus "treatment-as-usual" for behavior problems in children. Journal of Social Service Research 33:69–81. With 239 children; 83 SFT vs. 156 "treatment as usual". Better treatment engagement with SFT but no outcome differences. (jcorcoran@vcu.edu)

Franklin C., Moore K., Hopson L. (2008). Effectiveness of Solution-Focused Brief Therapy in a School Setting. Children and Schools 30(1):15–26. With 30 exp. (School A); 5–7 groups; 29 control (School B); 1-month follow-up (43). Teachers: externalised and internalised behaviours significantly improved; students externalised behaviours significantly improved.

Stith S. M., Rosen K. H., McCollum E. E., Thomsen C. J. (2004). Treating intimate partner violence within intact couple relationships: outcomes of multi-couple versus individual couple therapy. Journal of Marital and Family Therapy 30:305–318. With 14/20 individual couples, 16/22 multi-group couples completed the programme, 9 couples from the comparison group; all mild-to-moderate violence. Follow-up (women contacted): 6-month recidivism 43% individual, 25% multi-group, 67% comparison; 2-year recidivism: 0%, 13% (one client), and 50%. (Additional cases reported McCollum E. E., Stith S. M., Thomsen C. J. (2011). Solution-focused brief therapy in the conjoint couples treatment of intimate partner violence. Reduced physical aggression in both sexes for 17/20 individual couples; reduced in men only for 27/29 multi-group couples. In Franklin C., Trepper T., Gingerich W. J., McCollum E. (eds). Solution-focused Brief Therapy: A Handbook of Evidence-Based Practice. Oxford University Press: New York 2011.) (sstith@vt.edu)

Naturalistic studies (72) (only a few studies listed here)

Archuleta K. L., Burr E. A., Bell Carlson M., Ingram J., Irwin Kruger L., Grable J., Ford M. (2015). Solution Focused Financial Therapy: A Brief Report of a Pilot Study. Journal of Financial Therapy 6(1):2. http://dx.doi.org/10.4148/1944-9771.1081. Pilot study: solution-focused financial therapy client intervention approach. With eight college students: with a variety of financial issues related to budgeting, investing, and debt repayment problems. With a 3-month follow-up: psychological well-being and financial behaviours improved, financial distress decreased.

Beyebach M., Rodriguez Sanchez M. S., Arribas de Miguel J., Herrero de Vega M., Hernandez C., Rodriguez Morejon, A. (2000). Outcome of solution-focused therapy at a university family therapy center. Journal of Systemic Therapies 19:116–128. With 83 cases; telephone follow-up, most 1 year +. 82% satisfied; better outcome for "individual" problems than for "relational" ones; more dropout for trainees; with an average of 4.7 sessions (mark. beyebach@upsa.es)

Dumciene A., Rakauskiene V. (2014). Encouragement of Physical Activity among Students by Employing Short-term Educational Counselling. Procedia-Social and Behavioral Sciences 116:1523–152. http://dx.doi.

org/10.1016/j.sbspro.2014.01.428. With 92 students; after sf counselling, 44.6% previously facing physical activity issues achieved significantly positive changes, 21.7% achieved medium changes; and 33.7% showed minor changes. Physical activity increased, $p < 0.05$.

Fadilah N., Setiawati D. (2015). Application solution brief focused therapy (sfbt) to improve disclosure of self in Class VIII SMPN 1 Prambon. Journal BK UNESA 5(3). With five junior high school; low self-disclosure; improved significantly post-test after sf counselling. (nurfadillah994@ymail.com) (Indonesian)

Macdonald A. J. (2005). Brief therapy in adult psychiatry: results from 15 years of practice. Journal of Family Therapy 27:65–75. Additional 41 cases reported; with a 1-year follow-up. With 31 (76%) improved; with an average of 5.02 sessions; 20% single sessions. Combined total 118; 83 (70%) improved; and with an average of 4.03 sessions; 25% single sessions. Fewer new problems in the good outcome group. Longstanding problems predict less improvement; equal outcomes for all social classes.

Shennan G., Iveson C. (2011). From Solution to Description: Practice and Research in Tandem. In Franklin C., Trepper T., Gingerich W. J., McCollum E. (eds). Solution-focused Brief Therapy: A Handbook of Evidence-Based Practice. Oxford University Press: New York 2011.

With four studies. 24 clients, with a 6-month to 1-year follow-up: 23 (83%), better; 1 (3%), worse. With 39 clients, with an average of an 18-month follow-up: 31 (80%), better; 2 (5%). worse. With 57 clients with a 2–3-year follow-up: 24 (59.7%), improved; 2 (3.5%), worse. With 25 clients, with an 8—16-month follow-up: "best hopes" achieved by 14 (56%); little, 7 (28%); and not at all, 4 (16%).

Wiseman S. (2003). Brief intervention: reducing the repetition of deliberate self-harm. Nursing Times 99: 34–36. First self-harm 40 clients; one session. Up to a 6-month follow-up: 39 (97%) no repeat; 78% improved on self-scaling.

Yang Jee-Won, Kim Hyung-Mo (2015). A Research on the Effects of Solution-focused Group Art (2015) A Research on the Effects of Solution-focused Group Art Therapy on Improvement of Sibling Relationship and Well-being. South Korea Art Psychotherapy Association Article XIV:29.11(1):147–176. www.earticle.net/article. aspx?sn=244197. With six siblings: ten sessions group art therapy. Positive effects on sibling relationship, gentleness, conflict, relative status, competition, and the well-being of sibling children. (Korean)

Other resources (only a few studies listed here)

Franklin C., Trepper T. S., Gingerich W. J., McCollum E. (eds). Solution-focused Brief Therapy: A Handbook of Evidence-Based Practice. Oxford University Press: New York 2011.

A Comprehensive Review of the Evidence for the Effectiveness of SFBT (2013–2024) highlighted the following research papers:

Żak, A. M., & Pękala, K. (2024). *Effectiveness of solution-focused brief therapy: An umbrella review of systematic reviews and meta-analyses.* Psychotherapy Research, 1–13. https://doi.org/10.1080/10503307.2024.2406540

Vermeulen-Oskam, A., et al. (2024). *The current evidence of Solution-Focused Brief Therapy: A meta-analysis of psychosocial outcomes and moderating factors.* Journal of Counseling Psychology, 71(1), 23-45.

Neipp, M. C., & Beyebach, M. (2022). *The global outcomes of Solution-Focused Brief Therapy: A revision.* Psychotherapy Research, 32(2), 220-235.

Franklin, C., Zhang, A., Froerer, A., & Johnson, S. (2017). *Solution-focused brief therapy: A systematic review and meta-summary of process research.* Journal of marital and family therapy, 43(1), 16-30.

Zhang, X., et al. (2018). *The effectiveness of strength-based, Solution-Focused Brief Therapy in medical settings: A systematic review and meta-analysis of randomized controlled trials.* Journal of Behavioral Medicine, 41(5), 641-658.

Kim, J. S., Brook, J., & Akin, B. (2018). *Solution-Focused Brief Therapy with substance-using individuals: A randomized controlled trial study.* Substance Use & Misuse, 53(4), 583-592.

Moody, G., et al. (2024). *Solutions Trial: Solution-Focused Brief Therapy (SFBT) in 10–17-year-olds presenting at police custody: A randomized controlled trial.* Trials, 25(1), 159.

Mirghafourvand, M., Charandabi, S. M. A., Nahaee, J., & Rahmani, A. (2021). *The effect of Solution-Focused counseling on violence rate and quality of life among pregnant women at risk of domestic violence: A randomized controlled trial.* BMC Pregnancy and Childbirth, 21(1), 1-9.

González Suitt, J., & Franklin, C. (2021). *Evaluating the impact of Solution-Focused Brief Therapy on hope and clinical symptoms with Latin clients.* Journal of Ethnic & Cultural Diversity in Social Work, 30(1-2), 45-62.

Medina, A., Beyebach, M., & García, F. E. (2022). *Effectiveness and cost-effectiveness of a solution-focused intervention in child protection services.* Children and Youth Services Review, 143, 106703. https://doi.org/10.1016/j.childyouth.2022.106703

Lin, Y., & Chan, H. (2022). *Solution-focused coaching to improve medication adherence: A randomized controlled trial.* Patient Education and Counseling, 105(5), 1208–1214. https://doi.org/10.1016/j.pec.2021.09.014

Gan, C. (2020). *Solution-focused brief therapy (SFBT) with individuals with brain injury and their families.* NeuroRehabilitation, 47(1), 87–97. https://doi.org/10.3233/NRE-203001

Aminnasab, S., et al. (2018). *Effectiveness of solution-focused brief therapy on depression and perceived stress in patients with breast cancer.* Tanaffos, 17(4), 247–252. https://pubmed.ncbi.nlm.nih.gov/31143218/

Zhang, M., et al. (2021). *Effect of solution-focused brief therapy on cancer-related fatigue in patients undergoing chemotherapy: A randomized controlled trial.* Translational Cancer Research, 10(1), 371–380. https://doi.org/10.21037/tcr-20-2873

Franklin, C., et al. (2023). *Solution-focused brief therapy in schools: A review of research and practice.* School Social Work Journal, 47(2), 123–140.

Ramos-Heinrichs, P. (2023). *Empowering students who stutter: A solution-focused brief therapy approach.* Journal of Communication Disorders, 95, 105171. https://doi.org/10.1016/j.jcomdis.2023.105171

Taylor, C., & Biggs, H. (2017). *Utilizing solution-focused brief therapy with families living with autism spectrum disorder.*

Contemporary Family Therapy, 39(1), 12–20. https://doi.org/10.1007/s10591-017-9414-3

Ferraioli, S. J., & Hansford, A. (2019). *A pilot clinical outcome study of a parent training program for parents of children with autism spectrum disorder*. Autism Research and Treatment, 2019, 1–10. https://doi.org/10.1155/2019/5320714

Schleider, J. L., & Weisz, J. R. (2017). *Single-session digital interventions for youth: Advances and opportunities*. Annual Review of Clinical Psychology, 13, 149–177. https://doi.org/10.1146/annurev-clinpsy-032816-045214

Franklin, C., & Hai, A. H. (2021). *Brief intervention strategies for addressing workplace substance use: A solution-focused approach*. Journal of Occupational Health Psychology, 26(4), 517–529. https://doi.org/10.1037/ocp0000292

Bibliography

Aftab, A. (2020). Moving Beyond Psychiatric Diagnosis: Lucy Johnstone, PsyD. *Psychiatric Times*, August 14, 2020.

Bannink, F. (2014). *Post Traumatic Success: Positive Psychology & Solution-Focused strategies to help clients survive and thrive.* New York: Norton.

Bannink, F. (2016). *1001 Solution-Focused Questions.* New York: Norton.

British National Formulary (BNF). (2025). *British National Formulary (BNF89) March–September 2025: The First Choice for Concise Medicines Information.* London: Pharmaceutical Press.

Dolan, Y. (1991). *Resolving Sexual Abuse: Solution Focused Therapy & Ericksonian Hypnosis for Adult Survivors.* New York: Norton.

Dolan, Y. (1998). *Beyond Survival: Living Well is the Best Revenge.* London: BT Press.

Dolan, Y. and Johnson, C. (1995). In Dolan, Y. (1998), *Beyond Survival: Living Well is the Best Revenge.* London: BT Press.

DSM-V. (2013). *The Diagnostic and Statistical Manual of Mental Disorders.* Fifth Edition. Washington: American Psychiatric Association.

Erickson, M. H. In Haley, J. (1973). *Uncommon Therapy: The Psychiatric Techniques of Milton H. Erickson.* First Edition. New York: Norton.

Frankl, V. E. (1959). *From Death-Camp to Existentialism:* Boston: Beacon Press.

Frankl, V. E. (1960). Paradoxical Intention: A Logotherapeutic Approach. *American Journal of Psychotherapy,* **14**, 520–535.

Frankl, V. E. (1963). Experience with the Logotherapeutic Technique of Paradoxical Intention in the Treatment of Phobic and Obsessive-Compulsive Patients. (Paper read at the *Symposium of Logotherapy at the 6th International Congress of Psychotherapy,* London, UK, August 1964) *American Journal of Psychiatry,* **CXX 111**, No. 5 (1966), 548–553.

Frankl, V. E. (1964). *Man's Search for Meaning: An Introduction to Logotherapy.* London: Hodder & Stoughton.

Frankl, V. E. (1973). *The Doctor and the Soul: From Psychotherapy to Logotherapy.* Harmondsworth: Pelican Books.

Frankl, V. E. (1976). *Psychotherapy & Existentialism: Selected Papers on Logotherapy.* Harmondsworth: Pelican Books.

Frankl, V. E. (1978). *The Unheard Cry for Meaning.* London: Hodder & Stoughton.

Franklin, C., Trepper, T.S., Gingerich, W. J., and McCollum, E.E. (2012) *Solution-Focused Brief Therapy: a handbook of evidence-based practice.* Oxford University Press: New York.

Gardner, Frank. (2017). Frank Gardner: BBC Security Correspondent, Journalist and Author. http://www. frankgardner. co.uk/ (accessed 22 May 2017).

Gøtzsche, P. C. (2013). *How Big Pharma and Organized Crime has Corrupted Healthcare.* London: Radcliffe.

Griffin, J. and Tyrrell, I. (2004). *Human Givens: A New Approach to Emotional Health and Clear Thinking.* Delhi: H. G. Publishing.

Henden, J. (2011). *Beating Combat Stress: 101 Techniques for Recovery.* Hoboken, NJ: Wiley-Blackwell.

Henden, J. (2017). *Preventing Suicide: The Solution Focused Approach.* Second Edition. Hoboken, NJ: Wiley-Blackwell.

Hines, K. (2013). *Cracked, not Broken: Surviving and Thriving.* Lanham: Rowman & Littlefield Publishers.

Hines, K. (2014). The Kevin Hines Story. https://www.youtube.com/watch?v=loiGNZTfu6g (accessed 22 May 2017).

Hines, K. (2015). I Jumped off The Golden Gate Bridge. https://www.youtube.com/watch?v=WcSUs9iZv-g (accessed 22 May 2017).

Hines, K. (2017). The Kevin Hines Story. www.kevinhinesstory.com (accessed 22 May 2017).

Ivanov, I. and Schwartz, J. M. (2021). Why Psychotropic Drugs Don't Cure Mental Illness—But Should They? *Frontiers in Psychiatry*, **12**, 579566. https://doi.org/10.3389/fpsyt.2021.579566

Jacob, F. (2001). *Solution Focused Recovery from Eating Distress.* London: BT Press.

Johnstone, L. (2020). Why Mental Health Diagnoses Don't Work. https://www.youtube.com/watch?v=30FYlkOAwIE (accessed 13 September 2025).

Rothschild, B. (2000). *The Body Remembers: The Psychophysiology of Trauma and Trauma Treatment.* New York: Norton.

Sittser, J. L. (2009). *A Grace Disguised: How the Soul Grows Through Loss.* Grand Rapids: Zondervan.

Studio 10. (2017). Suicide Survivor Kevin Hines. https://www.youtube.com/watch?v=2XY96V13QbM (accessed 22 May 2017).

Vujicic, N. (2010). *Life without Limits: Inspiration for a Ridiculously Good Life.* New York: Crown Publishing Group.

Vujicic, N. (2012). No Arms, No Legs, No Problem. Promotional DVD for young people. www.youtube.com/watch?v=JpnMNzQKXaQQ (accessed 22 May 2017).

Vujicic, N. (2012). *Your Life without Limits.* New York: Crown Publishing Group.

Vujicic, N. (2013). *Limitless: Devotions for a Ridiculously Good Life.* New York: Crown Publishing Group.

Vujicic, N. (2013). *Unstoppable: The Incredible Power of Faith in Action.* New York: Crown Publishing Group.

Vujicic, N. (2014). *The Power of Unstoppable Faith.* New York: Crown Publishing Group.

Vujicic, N. (2015). *Stand Strong: You can Overcome Bullying (and Other Stuff that Keeps You Down).* New York: Crown Publishing Group.

Vujicic, N. (2016). *Love Without Limits. A Remarkable Story of True Love Conquering All.* New York: Crown Publishing Group.

Vujicic, N. (2017). Life Without Limbs. www.lifewithoutlimbs.org (accessed 22 May 2017).

Weston, S. (2025). Simon Weston CBE—Official Website. www.simonweston.com (accessed 27 November 2025).

Wikipedia. (2025). Frank Gardner (journalist). https://en.wikipedia.org/wiki/Frank_Gardner_(journalist) (accessed 27 November 2025).

Wikipedia. (2025). Nicholas James Vujicic. https://en.wikipedia.org/wiki/NickVujicic (accessed 27 November 2025).

Wisegeek. What is the Diaphragm Muscle? www.wisegeek.com/what-is-the-diaphragm-muscle.htm (accessed 27 November 2025).

Index

5-a-day, 73

5 o'clock rule, 167–8

5-4-3-2-1 Method, 7, 101

7/11 breathing, 5, 6, 21, 97

acceptance, 154

acknowledgement, 154

affirm, 174

anger build-ups, ways to deal with, 57–63

antidepressants, 134

anxiety, xviii

armed robbery, 180

Bannink, F., 143

barbecues, 3

Benefits of SF trauma recovery work, 175–7

biochemical, 144

black humour, 25

blame, 39

blocks, 169

blocks to disclosing, 169, 169–71, 180

"Breathe it away", 5

Breathing, 5, 6, 21, 81–82

breathing, 7/11, 5, 6, 9, 56

buddy-aid, xvi, 151, 161

changing the mindset, 46–48

child abuse and neglect, 180

cognitive-behavioual therapy (CBT), xiv

collaboration, 153

compassion, 147

compliment, 151, 174

confronting the flashback head-on, 20

correct apportionment of blame, 154

counsellors, xii

death and carnage, xvii

deep empathy, 147, 174

degrimming/black humour, 24, 43

de Shazer, Steve, xxiii

"depression" label, 144

determined, 173

diagnostic labeling, 144

diaphragm, 5, 21

diaphragmatic breathing, 65

diet, 73

discloses, 154, 173

disclosing/divulging, 154, 180

disease, 143

disempowering, xxi, 49

disorder, 143

divulging, 153

Dolan, Yvonne, xxiii, 44, 45, 51, 79, 165

dream(s) for the future, 109, 121

drugs, 136–8

dual awareness, 15

DVD, 19

Emotionally abusive, 10

Empower, 48

enhanced potential, 164

Erickson, Milton, 18, 44

evaluation, 186–206

evidence, 186–206

externalise the problem, 48

eye movement desensitisation and reprocessing (EMDR), 22

fast forwarding the DVD (FFDVD), 94, 112–116

Fast forward the livestream of your life, 54–57

fear, xviii

fireworks, 16

flashbacks, 2, 10, 11

fluids, 73

Frankl, Viktor, 134

Gardner, Frank, 126–7

getting back to sleep, 97–104

getting off to sleep, 94–97

goals, 164

God, 127, 130, 140–141

"Going with what works", xviii, xix, xxvii

Golden Gate Bridge, 129

Gøtzsche, Peter C., 136

Griffin, Joe, 135, 144

Griffin & Tyrrell, 18, 137

guided fantasy, 99

guilt, xviii, 37–41

Hamilton, Bethany, 122–3

Helpful questions & statements, 157–60

Henden, John, 174

Higher power, 140–1

Hines, Kevin, 129–33

homicide, 154

hope; hopeful, 141, 147–9

#HopeHelpsHeal, 133

Hsu, Prof Wei-Su, i

humour, 10, 74

Identify the source, 9

"If only…" monster, 25, 48–50

immediacy, 184

interrupting, 174

Intimacy, 139

Ivanov & Schwartz, 136

Jacob, Frederike, 48

Jargon-free, xiii

Johnson, Charlie, 51

#KeepOnKeepingOn, 133
kinaesthetic visualisation, 19

lay workers, xii
Lelonkiewicz, Jace, i
"Let it go… Let it go… Let it go",
  53–54
Letter from the future, 44–46
#LifeIsAGift, 133
link statement, 115
living life to the full, 105–149
Loo, Caroline, i
Lows, the, xii

Macdonald, Dr Alasdair, i, xxiv, 186
meaning and purpose, 107, 133–6,
  181
medication, 161
Milwaukee Brief Therapy Centre, 51
mindfulness, 7
Minnitt, Joy, xxiv
Moncrieff, J., 144
muggings, 180

naming the trauma, 180
natural disasters, 180
near-death, xvii, 180
near-death experiences, xvii, 180
negative feelings & emotions, 162
Neuroscience, 144
NLP, 18
normalised, 154
not your fault, 154

optimistic, 141

"Park it… and move on", 52–53
pharmaceutical industry, 144
Physical fitness, 74
Pihlaja, John, i
Pills, 40
post-traumatic growth (PTG), 143
post-traumatic stress reaction (PTSR),
  143
post-traumatic success (PTS), 143
Power-threat-meaning-framework
  (PTMF), 142
preparing well for bed, 87–93
Prescott, David, i
Procter, Prof Harry, i, xxiv
Professional, 161
psychobabble-free, xiii
psychotherapists, xii, 136
psychotherapy, 162
PTSD label, 142–3, 152
purpose in life, xviii, 164

qualities, 109–112, 146

rainy day letter, 79–80
replaying the DVD later, 25, 26–36
research, 157, 186–208
resistance, minimized, 153
resources, 105, 158
retraumatisation, 173–4
reverse psychology, 74, 94
"reversing (or "shrinking"),
  technique" 11, 12–14

revictimisation, 173–4
rewind technique, 18
Richard Bandler, 18
road traffic crashes/incidents, 13, 180

Samaritans, 82
self-blame, self-blaming, 37, 162
self-confidence, 75, 153
self-esteem, 75, 153
self-healing, 154
self-help, 161
serotonin deficit theory, 144
severe trauma, 131
SF Feelings tank, 68–69
shame, xviii, 142
"Shrinking" (or "the reversing
    technique"), 18, 155
Sittser, Gerald L., 148
skills, 93, 109–112
sleep disturbance, 83–105
small steps, power of, 94, 119, 143–4
smell of pork, 3
soldier, 4
solution focused, 160, 180
solution-focused brief therapy
    (SFBT), xiv, xxii, 180
solution-focused feelings tank, 62,
    181
Solution Focused in Organisations
    (SFiO), xxvii
"Stop!" technique, 26–36
strength-based questions, 173
strengths, 106, 109, 157
sudden death, 180

suicide, 127, 154
support, 163
supportive people, 77
survivor guilt, 37–41
survivors, xi–xiii, xv–xvii, xxi, xxv,
    153–4, 161–4, 173–4
Symptom-alleviation, xvi
symptoms, 161
syndrome, 143

"Tackle the guilt trip", 37–41
telephone helplines, 163
"Tell it, don't bottle it", 41–43
terrorist attacks, 180
"That was then, this is NOW!", 2, 4
the authentic life, 108, 164–5
"the lows", 76, 77, 82
the rainy-day letter, 72, 79–80
therapy, vii, 153
threats to kill, 180
thriver, xxi, xxv, 161–4
"toolbox", xv
traumatic, 161, 162
traumatic brain injury, 109
traumatic incidents, 162
traumatic memories, 153
traumatise, xiii
triggers, xvii, 1–10
trusting relationship, 154
Two-day workshops, 179–183
Tyrrell, Ivan, 137

undeclared or unresolved issues, 144
unexpressed emotion, 144

unwelcome thoughts, 25–70, 63–64,
158

validation, 154
victims, xxi, 161–4
visualisation, 26, 64–68, 90, 96
Voluntarily, bring on a pleasant
flashback, 21

Welcoming Triggers Through
Mindfulness, 7
wellbeing, 163
Weston, Simon, 124–6
what works, xix
Wisegeek, 56
Wright, Alison, xxiv
"Write, read & burn", 51

Yousafzai, Malala, 123–4